PORD
2221
9/12/99
£13-99

D0244039

SPORTS MASSAGE

WB 8756810 1

SPORTS MASSAGE

Dr Jari Ylinen and Mel Cash

BILSTON COMMUNITY COLLEGE
RESOURCES SERVICE

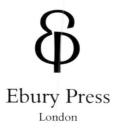

Ebury Press

London

BILSTON COMMUNITY COLLEGE
RESOURCES SERVICE

615.822 YLI | WR

4 DEC 1999 | 8756810

3 5 7 9 10 8 6 4 2

Copyright © Dr Jari Ylinen and Mel Cash 1988

Dr Jari Ylinen and Mel Cash have asserted their moral right
to be identified as the authors of this work in accordance
with the Copyright, Design and Patents Act 1988.

All rights reserved. No part of this publication may be
reproduced, stored in a retrieval system, or transmitted in
any form or by any means, electronic, mechanical,
photocopying or otherwise, without the prior permission of
the copyright owner.

First published in the United Kingdom
in 1988 by Stanley Paul.

This edition published in 1997 by

Ebury Press
Random House UK Ltd
Random House
20 Vauxhall Bridge Road
London SW1V 2SA

Random House Australia (Pty) Ltd
20 Alfred Street
Milsons Point Sydney
New South Wales 2016 Australia

Random House New Zealand Limited
18 Poland Road, Glanfield
Auckland 10 New Zealand

Random House South Africa (Pty) Limited
Endulini, 5A Jubilee Road
Parktown 2193, South Africa

Random House UK Limited Reg. No. 954009

A CIP catalogue record for this book is
available from the British Library.

ISBN 0 09 173746 X ✓ TB

Printed and bound in Great Britain by
Scotprint Ltd, Musselburgh, Scotland.

CONTENTS

ACKNOWLEDGEMENTS

The authors would like to express their thanks to the following people: Diane Mainzer for the illustrations, Keith Miller for the photography, Rael Isacowitz and Susan Nettleton for acting as models, and John Hands for his help and advice.

FOREWORD

Anybody competing in top-level sport constantly puts his or her body under stress, both in training to achieve peak performance and during competition. As in other sports, marathon running habitually works the body to the point of breakdown. Occasionally it may go beyond this, resulting in either an overuse or traumatic injury.

During eight years of competing in athletics for Great Britain, I have found that massage:

• assists recovery between intense training sessions

• monitors stresses which may be building up in the body, and so warns against potential injury

• is the most effective treatment for many types of injury

• helps recuperation after injury.

It is essential that sportsmen and women, coaches and masseurs are all continually aware of what parts of the body are put under exactly what kinds of stress by different sports and different types of training sessions. Massage treatment can then be much more effective in its employment, direction and results.

I have received massage treatment in Hungary, the United States and China as well as in Britain. It was only when I started having regular massage at the hands of Mel Cash that I had the treatment I was receiving adequately explained to me. I was impressed by the way that this enabled me to assist in directing the treatment to better overall effect.

I am pleased to see this explanation presented graphically and systematically in this book by Jari Ylinen and Mel Cash. I believe it is a major advance in matching massage treatment to the specific needs of sportsmen and women, and will prove invaluable for athletes, coaches and masseurs.

HUGH JONES

Hugh Jones is recognized as Britain's most consistent marathon runner. He has represented Great Britain at Olympic Games, European and World Athletic Championships since 1981. He won the London Marathon in 1982, and finished second in 1986 and third in 1987.

PREFACE

There have been many books written on massage, some of which are listed later in the bibliography, but to date there have been none covering the specific area of sports massage. This subject is of increasing importance, and not just for therapists who treat top competitive sportsmen. More people today are becoming concerned about health and are leading more active lives. People of all ages and from all walks of life are taking up sport and discovering the benefits on physical, psychological and social levels. Physical improvement usually encourages greater effort in training, and, without access to professional services and back-up, problems can develop. Competitive sportsmen push themselves to extreme limits and so have special needs which must be taken into account when preventing injuries and providing fine-tuning. Therapists need to understand the specific approach of sports massage so they can enable people to remain active and perform well.

Sports Massage is not only aimed at the therapist, but also at sportsmen who need to be aware of the effects of this therapy. Sportsmen often have to be their own treatment coordinators, and they can benefit by understanding the treatment they require. They should be able to give some basic self treatment. Coaches should be aware of the effects and uses of sports massage and maintain contact with the therapist. *Sports Massage* can offer valuable information not only on the sportsman's condition but also on the effects of training. This kind of monitoring is important for achieving optimal results and to avoid overuse injuries and traumas.

The type of injuries suffered by sportsmen do not differ from those in many other activities. If a muscle becomes strained, it matters little whether it is the result of digging in the garden, dancing in Swan Lake, or lifting weights in a gym. The damage to the tissues is the same and so are the principle massage techniques, but their application may be different. The massage techniques and advice in this book can be used for treating all soft tissue disorders. It is also important to know when massage should not be applied, so the contraindications are explained.

Sports Massage deals with the techniques and basic routines as well as the treatment of specific injuries which are related to various sports. Different sports have their own particular requirements; however, it would not be practical to describe complete massage routines for all individual sports as this would involve much repetition and run to several volumes. Such a list would, in fact, be misleading because people in the same sport may differ in training methods, performance standards, body type, and many other factors. The therapist treats the sportsman, not the sport.

We hope that this book will give information and guidance, not just to the student, but also to the experienced therapist. It is our wish that *Sports Massage* will promote effective massage treatment to become available to all, from top professionals to amateur and recreational sportsmen.

Jari Ylinen, MD, DO, Turku, Finland
Mel Cash, BA, LCSP(Assoc.), London, England

1
THE USE OF
MASSAGE IN SPORT

As sporting standards continue to improve, the intensity of training methods increases accordingly. Nowadays the amateur sportsman may train as much as the top professionals did a decade ago, but there is a price to be paid for such a high level of effort.

The body needs to rest to enable it to recover from the fatigue which results from hard training, and to enable it to develop the resilience necessary to achieve increased performance. As training builds up progressively a point is reached where the body is no longer able to fully recover between sessions, and performance may level off and eventually decline.

The symptoms of incomplete recovery are muscle pain, joint pain, tendon inflammation and bursa inflammation. Other indicators of this overtraining may include restlessness and difficulty in sleeping caused by physical tension and general aches and pains.

When the musculoskeletal system is being overtrained in this way it becomes vulnerable to trauma. Whilst following a seemingly normal training schedule one could suffer acute conditions like severe muscle strain, joint sprains and stress fractures. These in fact seldom happen by accident and can be avoided with a more comprehensive approach to recovery.

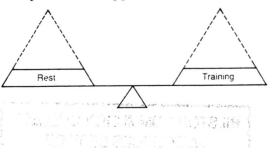

One must have enough rest time to allow the systems of the body to recover fully between training sessions. With only twenty-four hours in a day, and the increased training demands, full recovery may not be possible unless the effectiveness of the rest periods is improved.

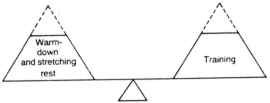

The importance of warming down and stretching is well understood and should be an integral part of a training programme. In spite of doing these exercises properly, however, there may still be local muscle tension preventing full recovery. Stretching tends to work the muscle groups as a whole, but the muscle does not work as a single unit in this way. It is divided into many sub-compartments, each of which work with different effort to produce the complexity of movement required. Also the normal range of movement in some joint restricts the effectiveness of stretching.

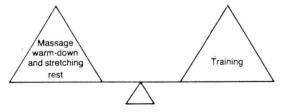

Massage can be used for the general relaxation of the musculo-skeletal system as well as being directed into local problem areas, thereby improving recovery and ensuring it happens thoroughly.

The sportsman should be aware of the uses and benefits of massage so he can make the best use of it. All sporting activities involve muscle activity as the primary motive force, and many sports injuries are directly muscle injuries or originate from muscle dysfunction. Massage is the best form of treatment for muscle tension, and has the distinct advantage over most other therapies in that it can be used on a regular basis to help prevent overuse injuries as well as being used as a symptom based approach to the treatment of specific injuries.

With massage the therapist can remove the accumulation of general aches and pains that some sportsmen either seem to accept as normal due to their gradual build-up, or try to suppress with drugs. These aches and pains can lead to more serious problems, so the benefits of massage for injury prevention are great. With specific injuries massage can explore the soft tissues more intimately than any other therapy, and problem areas can be diagnosed and treated very accurately. Mechanical massage machines and electrotherapy equipment, which are widely used today for treating sports injuries, are easier to use for the therapist, but they offer no direct feedback on the changes taking place in the tissues. With massage the therapist is acutely aware of these changes through the feeling in the hands and so can adapt the treatment accordingly. For this reason every treatment can be uniquely suited to the specific needs of the sportsman at that time.

BILSTON COMMUNITY COLLEGE
RESOURCES SERVICE

2
THE EFFECTS
OF SPORTS MASSAGE

FRICTION

Hands sliding along the skin cause friction which creates much of the heat derived from massage. Friction also occurs between all the tissue layers as they are moved against each other, which generates more heat. Some heat is formed by the opening of arteries and capillaries through pumping effect and axonal reflexes caused by massage stimulation. The improvement in the microcirculation brings more warming blood to superficial layers. The release of intracellular enzymes like histamine will also create some heat. These warming effects are beneficial as they increase the pliability of the tissues and improve the metabolism. Despite the many benefits of heat, it is not one of the main therapeutic benefits of massage, and it can be more easily obtained by other means like hot packs and saunas.

PUMPING

Every stroke made along the flow of the venous and lympathic systems assists their circulation. As massage is applied it causes increased pressure in the vessels in front of the stroke and a subsequent vacuum in those behind. Both these pressure changes assist the flow of fluid in the venous and lymphatic vessels and will make room for new fluids coming from deeper tissues. Increase in the return flow will obviously improve arterial blood supply which has to refill the cleared vessels. This does not have very significant benefits if the tissue is in good condition,

although there has been shown to be a measurable improvement in total blood-flow in the massaged parts. When muscles are tense or there is increased pressure in muscle compartments the circulation is inhibited, not only in the muscles, but also in other tissues like joints, ligaments and tendons. As blood is rich with oxygen and other substances vital for repair and growth, the pumping effect achieved with massage is essential to restore normal tissue condition.

INCREASED TISSUE PERMEABILITY

Deep stroking massage techniques create a localised increase in pressure, which causes the pores in tissue membranes to open, facilitating the exchange of fluids. It improves the removal of muscle waste like lactic acid, which builds up in the muscles during and immediately after hard exercise. The highly oxygenated fluids rich in nutrients are then absorbed more easily. This is necessary to normalise tissue metabolism and to facilitate the repair and build-up of tissues following training. As a result of increased tissue permeability one can measure the increase of tissue enzyme levels in the blood after massage.

STRETCHING

Sportsmen are aware of the importance of stretching, and massage techniques can also achieve stretching of muscles, tendons and fascia. In addition massage can stretch those other tissues that cannot be reached by any other method. There is a distinct difference between the stretching done by a sportsman and that achieved through massage. Normal stretching exercises treat the muscle, or more usually the muscle group, as a whole. As the stretch is performed the muscle attachments are drawn away from each other, causing the fibres to lengthen, and the muscle bundles are brought closer together. In massage muscle bundles are pulled longitudinally and are moved transversely. This both stretches the fibres and moves the bundles apart, thus improving intramuscular circulation and breaking possible adhesions between the muscle bundles. So, with massage the fibres can be stretched in all directions and not just in line with the attachments.

Massage has an advantage in that it can be used to stretch muscles regardless of joint range. The conventional type of stretching carried out by sportsmen is often restricted by the limitation of normal or restricted joint movement. Stretching with massage is always applied to localised areas and can be carried out systematically throughout the muscle. This makes it possible to regulate the amount of stretch applied to different parts depending on the relative tension found. With normal stretching the less tensile areas give way first and localised tight areas are stretched less.

With massage it is possible to apply stretching to specific structures like fascia (which surrounds the muscles) unlike normal stretching which affects all the structures in a general area equally. Stretching fascia through massage releases muscle tension. This is particularly important in cases of compartment syndrome where tense fascia causes increased intrafascial pressure.

BREAKING

Scar tissue may be present in soft tissues, like muscles, tendons and ligaments, of the sportsman as a result of past injuries or the gradual build-up of overuse injuries due to repeated microtrauma. This can cause tension and inflexibility, which may lead to local or referred problems. Adhesions may occur where fibrous tissue causes different tissues to stick together due to inflammation as well as microtrauma. This will reduce the tensile property of tissues and may restrict movement. Deep friction massage technique is used to break down scar tissue and adhesions. It will help the return of normal tissue tension, and will restore both contractile properties and a normal range of movement.

Fibrosis seldom affects whole muscles in sportsmen as it is a condition which tends to affect inactive muscles, but long-standing tension can imply localised inactivity which can lead to atrophy and fibrosis occurring in some sportsmen. It is often not apparent because it can affect only part of the muscle while other parts continue to work seemingly normally and can even compensate for it to some extent. The only symptoms may be long-standing diffused pain, tension and restricted movement. In sportsmen this condition is more likely to occur in the postural muscles, for example in the neck and back muscles. This is because these muscles work mainly isometrically. With massage one can apply an effective stretch on local areas of the muscle to relieve tension and, by cross friction, to break down fibrosis.

IMPROVED TISSUE ELASTICITY

Excessive repetitive and particularly long-standing isometric type of muscle effort makes tissues hard and inelastic. This causes the metabolism to suffer; normal tissues begin to waste and are slowly replaced by fibritic and less elastic components. This is why hard training does not necessarily improve performance and can even have a contradictory effect. By kneading soft tissues it is possible to pull the elastic structures to near their maximal length in all directions. This is necessary to maintain normal elasticity in tissues which are continually put under great stress in certain positions.

OPENING MICRO-CIRCULATION

Measurements have shown that massage increases total bloodflow through the treated part. This in itself is not significant as active exercises of the muscles increases total bloodflow much more. The important thing is that massage opens arterioles and capillaries, so improving the exchange of fluids to the tissues. Deep massage causes the release of vasoactive substances creating a dilation of the vessels which bring new fluid to the tissues. The size of the vessels is also controlled by the autonomous nervous system, and it is even possible to increase microcirculation with just superficial massage, through the reflexes.

PAIN REDUCTION

With intensive training one tends to get excessive muscle tension which restricts circulation and deprives the tissues of oxygen. Metabolic waste products accumulate in these tissues, which causes pain. This is particularly common where tight fascia surrounds the muscles and there is increased intrafascial pressure which further blocks the circulation. The mechanical effects of the massage will improve these conditions by increasing circulation and stretching as described in more detail above.

Long-standing restriction of movement because of pain, splinting, bad posture or other reasons causes the elastic component of soft tissues to shrink and form into inelastic fibrous tissues. Because of this, pain arises during normal movement. Again the stretching effects of massage are beneficial and result in relief of pain.

Massage is able to reduce pain by reflexes affecting the central nervous system. It causes the release of endorphins which abolish pain sensations in the brain. Stimulation of the mechanoreceptors by massage has been shown to reduce pain and muscle tension. According to 'gate control' theory this is because stimulation prevents pain impulses going beyond the dorsal horn of the spinal chord. Perception of pain is also modulated by sensory input to other parts of the central nervous system, especially the mid-brain. Acupressure therapy is a sophisticated method of eliminating pain and is explained in detail in a later chapter.

RELAXATION

Local relaxation of the muscles is achieved by many of the mechanical effects of massage, like increased warmth, circulation and stretching. Reflectory effects are sometimes even more important in achieving relaxation. Massage stimulates the mechanoreceptors, which sense touch, pressure, tissue length, movement and warmth in muscle and other connective tissues. Reflex pathways via the central nervous system transmit the stimulus and induce relaxation through efferent pathways to muscles.

Overall tension is dependent on total sensory input to the central nervous system. General relaxation is better achieved when a large area of the body is treated. This is reached in a combination of three different types of massage:

...General tension is maintained by local stiffness and aches which can be relieved with deep stroking massage techniques. When this has been resolved irritative impulses from problem areas will stop.

...One is able to create awareness of relaxation further by soft general massage.

...There are specific areas where massage causes relaxation as a reflectory response. This will be dealt with in the chapter on acupressure therapy.

BALANCING AUTONOMOUS NERVOUS SYSTEM

Reducing muscle tension and abolishing pain due to musculoskeletal disorders, especially in the neck, is shown to decrease the recurrence of migraine attacks, lowers high blood pressure and may stop hyperventilation syndrome. These effects achieved by massage are due to reduced output from irritated mechanoreceptors from muscles and tendons which causes sympathetic nervous system overactivity. This will also help get better relaxation and improves sleep after strenuous exercise. Massage eases abdominal pain in constipation by stimulating the parasympathetic nervous system and improving the mobility of the intestines. It may help to normalize bowel function which is disturbed due to psychological or physical stress.

Mechanical effects

friction warming
pumping the circulation
stretching soft tissue
breaking scar tissue
breaking adhesions
increased tissue permeability
opening microcirculation
enzyme release
improved tissue elasticity

Reflectory effects

relaxation
pain reduction
opening microcirculation
balancing autonomous nervous
   system

3
HOW TO GIVE GENERAL SPORTS MASSAGE

THE PLACE

Massage should ideally be carried out in a warm, quiet and well ventilated room, as this will create the right atmosphere for comfort and relaxation. The warmth of the room is important as cold increases muscle tension and will prevent relaxation. In practice, one may end up having to improvise from time to time and to work wherever the space can be found: by the side of the track, in the changing rooms or even in the broom cupboard. What is most important is the massage, not the fancy treatment room.

THE TREATMENT COUCH

An adjustable treatment couch with a face hole is the best thing to use for massage, because it enables the therapist to change the height depending on the size of the sportsman, the part of the body being treated and the amount of pressure required. Using a face hole in the prone lying position allows the muscles on both sides of the neck and shoulders to be in a relaxed position, so allowing the therapist to treat them more effectively. With a non-adjustable treatment couch the recommended height for sports massage is from the level between the lower and middle third of the thigh to the mid-thigh of the therapist. If the couch is too high one cannot use body weight properly to apply pressure, and this can lead to strain in the neck and shoulder muscles of the therapist. A couch set too low means the therapist has to bend more, which can cause problems in the lower back. One advantage of an adjustable couch is that one has to keep moving to work from different positions, which tends to prevent overuse of particular muscles. A portable couch is essential if it is necessary to work at different locations. There are both adjustable and non-adjustable portable couches available.

The advantage of a couch is that one can move freely around it to find the best possible position to work from. Using a bed is not a good idea as it is too low and the therapist can injure his own back by leaning over it. Also, one cannot work effectively in this way as the patient will sink into the bed as pressure is applied. Situations sometimes arise where there is no treatment couch available; in this case it is best to use the floor with a thin covering, like a blanket, over it. Working on the floor is not recommended for regular use as it can become very uncomfortable for the therapist.

CUSHIONS

Cushions can help improve comfort and so make the muscles more relaxed for effective massage. When the patient is lying in the prone position (face down) having a cushion under the ankle joint will relax the legs and prevent cramp in the calf and foot, which otherwise quite often disturbs the treatment. The patient may feel more comfortable with another cushion under the head. In the supine position (face up) a cushion under the knees will keep the legs and abdomen relaxed. The patient may also prefer one under the head.

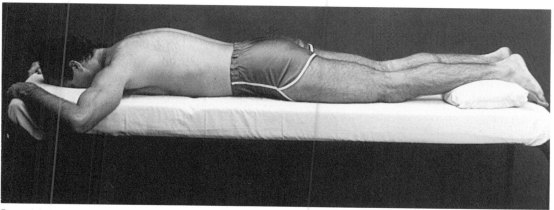

Prone lying position, using face hole and cushion under the ankles. A cushion may be used as a side support for the head, if there is no face hole. A cushion may be required under the stomach or under one side of the hip in cases of severe lower back pain

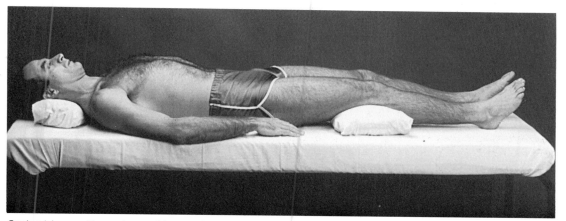

Supine lying position, using cushions under the head and knees to ensure maximal relaxation. A thin cushion may be required under the lower back in some cases of lower back pain

If there is no face hole on the couch a cushion can be used to support the head in a fairly straight position. Otherwise, lying in the prone position during half the treatment with the head turned sideways may cause tension in the neck and upper back.

Keeping the patient warm improves muscle relaxation, and it is very useful to use towels to cover the parts of the patient not being treated. It is especially important to cover the treated part after massage to maintain the heat that has been created. This will also prevent the chilling effect caused by oil evaporating on the skin.

LUBRICANTS

The therapist will need to use some kind of oil or cream as a lubricant to enable his hands to move smoothly over the skin and prevent pulling the patient's hair. (Dragging the hair is painful and quite often causes skin infections such as folliculitis.)

Soap solution has been used commonly before, but because of the increased heat conductivity and evaporation of the water it contains it cools the skin down quickly. Fine powder can be used to avoid skin traction, but it needs to be used liberally, which can prove very messy. There are many products on the market for massage, and it is a good idea to try some out to see what one is the best to work with. Massage oils often contain ingredients which stimulate circulation and have a warming effect. Sportsmen may feel comforted by this, but it may cause irritation on the hands of the therapist if used often. One should consider the safety of the ingredients when trying new oils, because some oil will always be absorbed through the skin. It is not really necessary to use an expensive product, any pure oil will do, for example baby oil, sunflower oil or olive oil. These usually suit people with allergies, which is an important point to consider. It is not good to use too much oil; it should be used little and often so as to maintain a degree of grip and control.

Massage can be done without any lubricants providing only short strokes are used, or if one is only working superficially or using just pressure techniques. This is sometimes more practical if time is short or if a localised area only is to be treated. However, increased skin friction must be taken into account. Lubricants are not helpful in pre-manipulative treatment as a manipulative therapist needs to have good grip on the skin to enable him to work effectively; and this is not possible if oil is present as it makes the skin slippery.

HEAT/ICE

Many therapists are accustomed to applying heat, either radiated from lamps or by direct contact with hot packs, before starting to massage. This is to soften and relax the muscles, and, although it is fairly effective, the same results will normally be achieved during the first few minutes of massage anyway. Heat is not always beneficial as initial treatment as it can sometimes make tissues more tender, particularly if there is fresh inflammation.

When treating specific areas which are acutely tender it may be nearly impossible to apply massage. One can start with very light gentle massage, gradually increasing the pressure as the sportsman becomes accustomed to it and the muscles gradually soften. This can be a slow process, taking many sessions to get effective results. If ice is applied to the area for a few minutes it can produce effective analgesia and will also relax the muscles. Proper massage may then be possible with effective results in the first session and subsequent treatments may not require the use of ice at all.

4
GENERAL MASSAGE TECHNIQUES

GENERAL HINTS

When giving massage, stand with your feet comfortably apart to maintain good balance. Keep your back straight to avoid unnecessary strain. Stand as close to the couch as possible. There will be times when you need to apply considerable pressure in an effort to achieve good results with muscle tension. To do this you should use your body weight rather than arm strength, otherwise you may be exhausted before finishing your first massage.

Below left: Correct standing position for the therapist: maintaining normal lower back lordosis even when leaning forwards, and using the weight of the whole body to exert pressure and movement

Below right: Incorrect standing position for the therapist: by allowing the lower back muscles to relax, the normal lumbar curve is lost. The back is curved forwards and subject to excessive strain. If the arms are bent too much the therapist cannot use body weight to exert force and must work much harder with arms, causing fatigue and creating tension in the neck and shoulders

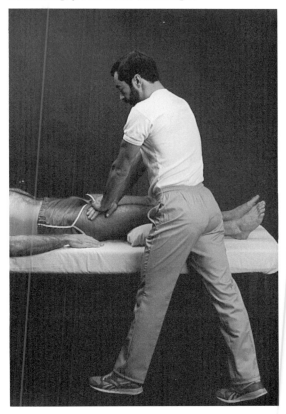 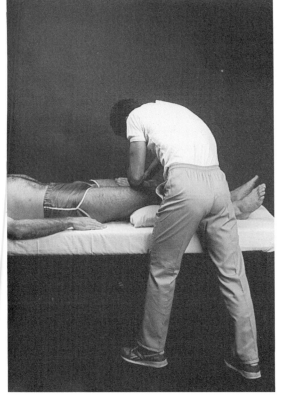

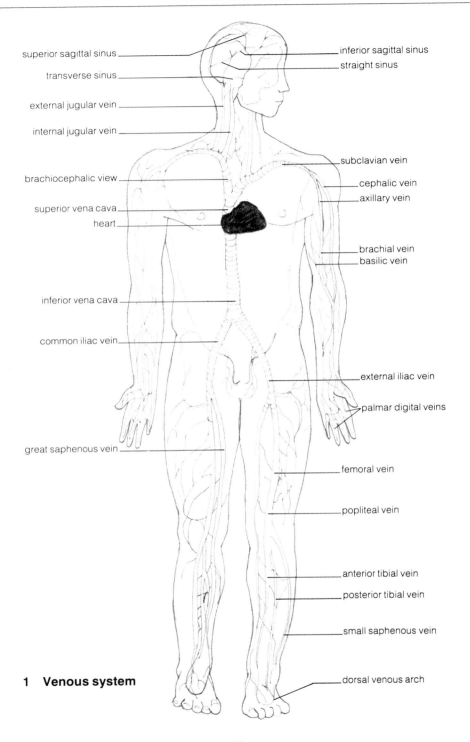

superior sagittal sinus

inferior sagittal sinus

straight sinus

transverse sinus

external jugular vein

internal jugular vein

subclavian vein

brachiocephalic view

cephalic vein

axillary vein

superior vena cava

heart

brachial vein

basilic vein

inferior vena cava

common iliac vein

external iliac vein

palmar digital veins

great saphenous vein

femoral vein

popliteal vein

anterior tibial vein

posterior tibial vein

small saphenous vein

dorsal venous arch

1   Venous system

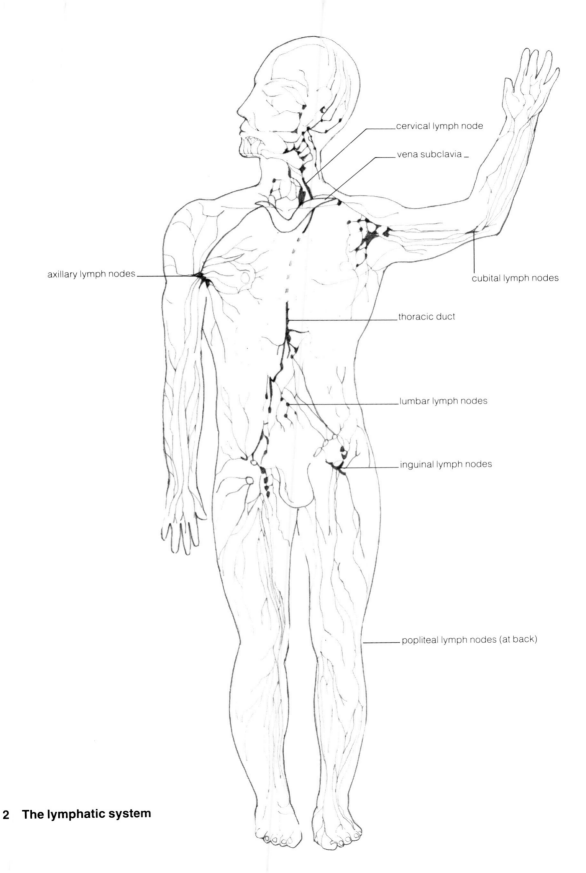

cervical lymph node

vena subclavia

cubital lymph nodes

axillary lymph nodes

thoracic duct

lumbar lymph nodes

inguinal lymph nodes

popliteal lymph nodes (at back)

2   The lymphatic system

When using massage oil you need to get the amount right. Too much, and you lose grip and control; too little, and you can cause skin soreness and possible infection. You will also find that some massage techniques can be done better with less oil on the skin than others. The best thing is to have the oil close to hand and in an easy to use dispenser; this way you can use it 'little and often'. Put the oil on your palms first and rub your hands together to warm it up before starting the massage. It is important that the first contact creates the right impression of confidence and ability. If trust is lost at the beginning it is very difficult to develop later.

DIRECTION OF MASSAGE

Massage should be directed towards the heart when treating the extremities to assist lymphatic and venous flow, which remove the waste product from the tissues. This will make the recovery process more effective and will shorten the time necessary for rest. If the massage pressure is applied in the opposite direction the valves of lymphatic vessels and superficial veins could become damaged. Movements in the opposite direction are possible only where short strokes are applied near the muscle attachments at the extremities.

The direction of the massage of the trunk is determined purely on the most effective way of applying the strokes and the condition being treated. There is no need to consider the direction of the circulation. However, massage should not be performed in just a longitudinal direction along the soft tissues, nor should it only be in a transverse direction. The most effective way to apply massage is with a combination of different techniques.

SUPERFICIAL STROKING (Effleurage)

This is a gentle stroking movement applied with the whole hand with the fingers

Opposite above: Superficial stroking: long strokes applied lightly on the legs using the whole hands. Performed in the direction of the heart. The whole body of the therapist should move and not just the arms

Opposite below: Superficial stroking: returning to the starting position of the stroke should be carried out by maintaining only light contact with the body

together or with the palm to cover a large surface area. Use a smooth, flowing and rhythmical action, with the hand forming to the contours of the muscles. Apply long strokes to cover a whole part, and use one hand or both hands side by side to cover a larger area. One hand at a time can be used alternately in a rhythmical way. Try to maintain contact with the skin at all times, so apply the main stroke in the direction of the venous and lymphatic flow, and then return by just sliding the hands back without any pressure.

Gradually increase the pressure as you apply the technique before using deep stroking. The most effective way of doing this is by placing one hand on top of the other, keeping the arms almost straight and using your body weight.

Superficial stroking is the first basic technique and should be used at the start of the treatment to spread the oil, warm the area, relax the muscles and acclimatise the

Superficial stroking of the arm using the thumb, index finger and/or the web between them

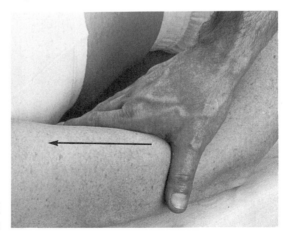

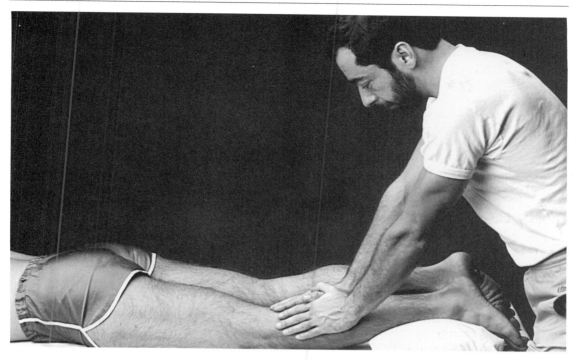

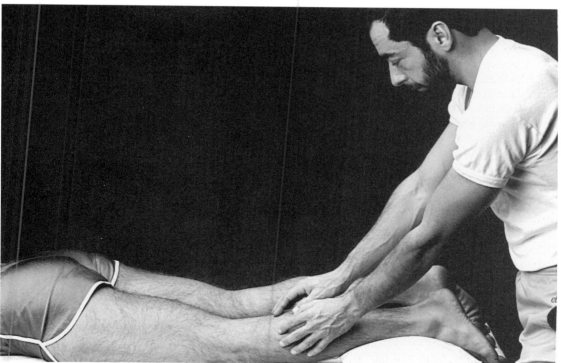

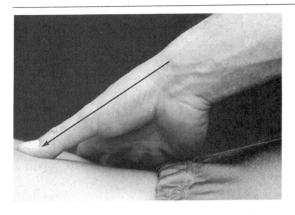

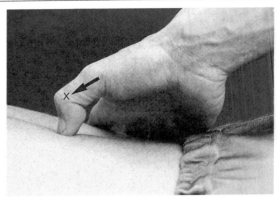

Correct use of the pad of the thumb: the bones of the thumb and arm are in line and the force is exerted straight along it

Incorrect position of the thumb: the bent thumb causes forced angular leverage on its joints inducing strain and arthritis. This will gradually lead to painful conditions and deformity of the thumb

patient. It is also a good technique for identifying general areas of tension which will require special attention. It should be returned to several times during treatment to maintain the relaxation, particularly after using some of the more specific deep techniques which may cause some pain. Use it to finish off the massage to leave a good level of relaxation.

DEEP STROKING

This is done using smaller surfaces of the hand to concentrate the pressure, or larger areas using considerable force:

Pad of the thumb
Pads of the fingers
Ulnar surface of the fist
Ulnar border of the palm
Heel of the palm
Ulnar border of the forearm
Elbow

Longitudinal stroking

Apply deep pressure and then make short strokes of two or three inches at a time. Begin each stroke by overlapping the previous one. Work systematically through the whole muscle in this way. It may be easier to treat large muscles in a few sections.

Strokes should be applied in the direction of the muscle fibres, which requires a good working knowledge of muscle anatomy. It is important to include the tendons and attachments and not just to treat the belly of the muscle. Near the attachment the direction of the strokes should be towards the belly of the muscle to apply a stretch to the tendons and induce a reflectory relaxation of the muscle. Try to treat each muscle individually, and also try to dig between muscles to help separate them. The deep stroking routine should be repeated several times with gradually increased pressure.

Where there is muscle tension this technique will not be painless. To get the most benefit use as much pressure as possible within the limit of excessive pain and avoiding muscle contraction. For this reason conduct the strokes much slower and with more care than in superficial stroking. Successful massage can of course be achieved painlessly, but it could take several sessions to get the same results.

Deep longitudinal stroking is a very important technique in sports massage and is most effective when applied to particularly tense muscles. It is the best

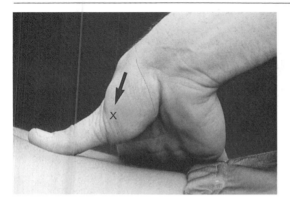

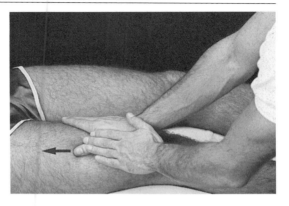

Incorrect position of the thumb: the extended thumb causes forced angular leverage on its joints inducing strain and arthritis

The thumb used as a tool with the other hand pressing down on it and moving it

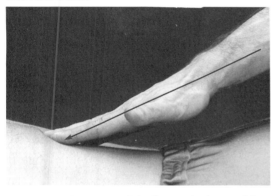

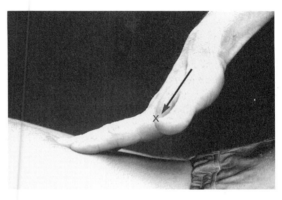

Correct use of the pads of the fingers: the bones of the fingers, hand and arm are in the same line. The force is exerted straight to the fingertips

Incorrect position of the fingers: the bent fingers cause angular leverage inducing strain and arthritis to joints of the fingers

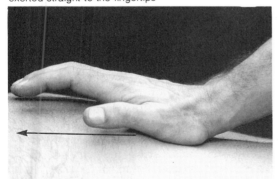

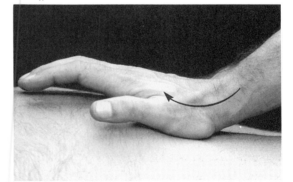

Above left: Correct use of the heel of the palm: longitudinal strokes are performed with the wrist kept at a fixed angle. *Above right:* Incorrect use the heel of the palm: making a habit of rolling the wrist during strokes quickly causes aching and induces arthritis to joints of the wrist. This is because during the rolling movement the bones of the wrist move in relation to each other while a strong compression force is also effecting them. Instead, similar rolling movements can be made without strain by lifting and lowering the elbow while the wrist is kept locked

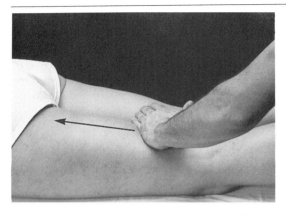

Using the ulnar border of the hand for massage. This is a fairly large smooth area and the effect is acquired mainly by compression

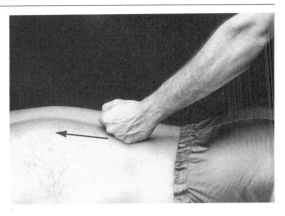

Using the ulnar border of the fist for massage

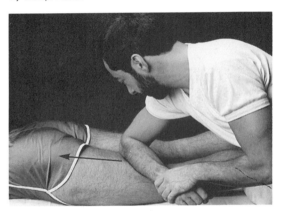

Using the ulnar border of the forearm

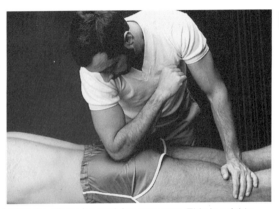

Using the elbow for applying massage. This is a fairly insensitive part and great force is easily generated. It should only be used in special cases when extra force is needed

technique for stretching the muscle as it can work on small areas which are affected by local tension. In so doing it also induces deep relaxation and is good at removing muscle waste.

Transverse stroking

Grasp across the belly of the muscle using the flat of the hands. Using the thumb or the heel of the palm as an anchor point, draw the fingers towards it moving deeply through the muscle and allowing it to flow under your finger tips. This is often done the other way around using the fingers as a fixed point pressing them down, or just lying on the skin, with the palm moving towards it, allowing the soft tissues to pass under. Areas not accessible to the whole hand can be treated with the pads of the fingers, reinforced with the other hand bearing down on them. Any bands of local muscle tension will become noticeable as it will not pass smoothly under the fingers.

This is primarily a diagnostic technique, but it can also be used to separate the

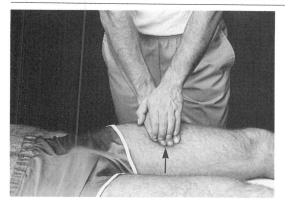

Deep transverse stroking using the fingertips with the force being strengthened by the other hand

bands of muscle from each other and also away from the bone by stretching the tight areas laterally.

KNEADING (Petrissage)

This is usually applied with both hands in a rhythmical way. Using the whole hand, grasp, lift and release a muscle or muscle group with alternate hands. They should work together in the same way as if kneading dough. Of course one should avoid pinching the skin or digging in with the finger tips.

Kneading is not really suited for tense

Kneading: both hands working alternately, gripping and releasing the muscle in a rhythmical way. Left hand grasping and right hand releasing in this picture

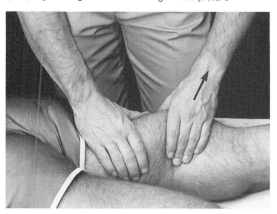

muscles because it is very irritating if the muscle is not sufficiently pliable. On soft muscles it helps pump the circulation of blood and tissue fluids so speeding up recovery. The kneading action tends to create movement between muscle bands so improving elasticity and flexibility.

SQUEEZING

Grasp the muscle or muscle group with both hands and squeeze: push both hands across the direction of the muscle to stretch it sideways; then push and pull with alternate hands causing cross stretching of the fibres between the hands.

Squeezing: using both hands simultaneously to grip the muscle between thumb and fingers. Stretch the muscle in the same direction with both hands

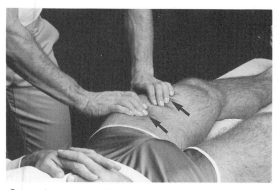

Squeezing: using both hands simultaneously to grip and stretch the muscle in opposite directions

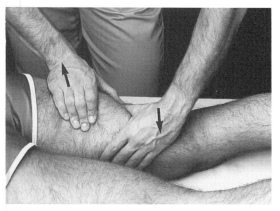

These techniques create transverse movement between the deep layers of muscle tissue, different muscles and between muscles and bones. This should always be included in sports massage because other techniques do not reach the tissue so deeply.

DEEP FRICTION

Apply this technique with the pads of your thumb or finger tips. Greater pressure can be applied by the forefinger over the middle finger. The greatest force can be applied by using fingers of one hand as a passive tool with the power coming from the other hand bearing down on it.

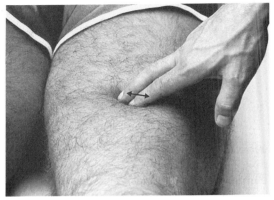

Deep friction, using the tip of the middle finger reinforced by the index finger to apply deep pressure with back and forth or rotational movements across lesions

It is applied only on local problem areas such as scar tissue and hard bands of muscle which are the result of overuse and injuries. Press deeply into these areas, within pain tolerance, and give a slow frictional movement in a transverse direction against the muscle fibres and/or a circular direction. This will cause considerable pain, and it is advisable to warn the sportsman first and explain why it needs to be done. It is important that the patient does not tense up to resist the pain but to actually try to relax into it.

Friction can be applied around joints to break down any fibrosis formed in traumatised ligaments and to stimulate circulation. In many cases of muscle tension, tenderness is found at the musclotendinous junction. This is where strains and scar tissue most commonly occur because the tissues are more compact and there is less movement between the fibres.

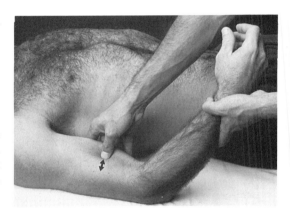

Deep friction, using the thumb

Deep friction breaks down scar tissue, which is inelastic, and restricts movement of tendons as well as efficient muscle contraction. After joint sprains, damaged ligaments repair by forming new fibrous tissue. This can be hard, inelastic and less resilient, especially if the joint has been immobilised. By applying deep friction massage one hinders this build up of scar tissue and promotes the formation of more tolerable elastic fibrous tissue. Scar tissue is one of the main causes of long term painful conditions, and as it also affects function it can cause other injuries. Hard bands of muscle fibres occur where the scar tissue from microscopic muscle damage causes fibres to adhere together preventing their independent movement. The deep friction releases these adhesions. It also has the effect of stimulating the local blood supply to such problem areas, thus promoting healing.

28

DEEP PRESSURE

This is normally applied using the thumb or the middle finger supported by the forefinger. Tender points can usually be found whilst applying deep stroking techniques. They are located in skin, scar tissue, fascia, muscles, tendons, ligaments, joint capsules and periosteum.

When a point has been found, apply pressure to it, increasing gradually till a maximum pain tolerance has been reached. There are conflicting views on how long this pressure should be held for, ranging from a few seconds to several minutes. The best results are found when it is held until

Deep pressure or small rotations applied with the thumb on local tender points of the upper arm. Pressure should be increased gradually to avoid excessive pain until a maximum is reached within pain tolerance. Pressure is released when the tissue becomes insensitive or relaxation of the muscle is achieved

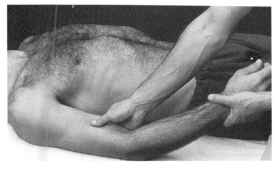

Deep pressure applied with the fingers on local tender area of the arm (lung channel see acupressure therapy)

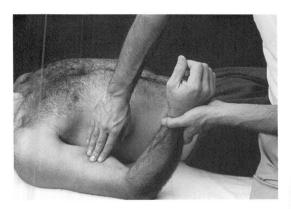

there is a significant reduction in pain, so it depends on each individual case. Some therapists use further stimulation by applying a rotational movement to the point while simultaneously pressing. When pain is caused in the area around the point or referred to other parts by stimulation these tender points are called trigger points. These will be dealt with in detail in a later chapter. With muscle tension, tenderness is often experienced at the ends of the muscle. By irritating these tender points with deep pressure one causes a reflex action with the central nervous system which encourages local muscle relaxation – neuro-muscular technique (or NMT). These deep frictions should be applied for only one second at a time as they cause a very sharp pain and to sustain them for any longer would be intolerable.

PERCUSSION (Tapotement)

These are techniques using both hands alternately, working very quickly and rhythmically. There is a wide variety of applications including clapping, hacking and beating.

These techniques are not relaxing; on the contrary they are to stimulate muscles. They should not be used on traumatised muscles, and are really only of use in preparing the muscles for competition. The general excitement and race preparation usually provides the sportsman with sufficient stimulation, so percussion is rarely necessary. It is useful, however, in maintaining muscle tone and preventing unwanted relaxation during short rest breaks in competition such as those between heats and the final. It is often used on people involved in contact sports as it heightens muscle tone and so improves resilience to impact.

29

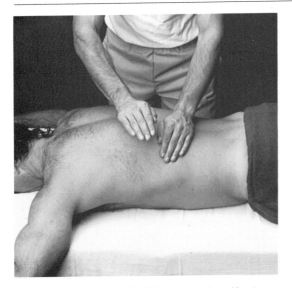

Clapping: the hands are held in a cupped position to cause a pocket of air to be made with the skin. There should be no slapping. The quick repetitive clapping movements are made mainly from the elbow

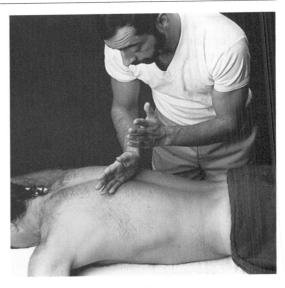

Hacking: with the fingers slightly spread and relaxed so a vibration effect is experienced when they strike the surface

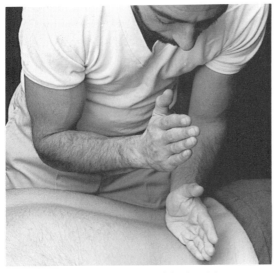

Hacking: using the ulnar border of the hand for a more penetrating effect

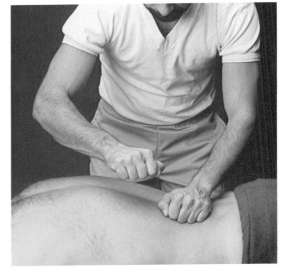

Beating: a rapid striking of the skin using the palmar aspect of the fist

SHAKING

This is applied by using one or both hands to gently grasp the muscle towards its ends and to loosely shake the muscle with small amplitude from side to side. Sometimes it is beneficial to apply the technique to a whole part of the body by grasping the hand or foot and introducing movement up and down or sideways. Shaking is a useful technique to be applied between deep massage sessions when the sportsman may tense up. It is also particularly good as a closing movement to finish the massage, as it leaves a good feeling of relaxation.

VIBRATION

A vibration movement can be applied using the hand or the fingers, depending on the size of the area being stimulated. Some therapists use it for the stimulation of acupuncture points and channels. When applied to a small area it causes irritation, and a reflectory response results. When using slight pressure of the hand it promotes relaxation. The effects of mechanical massage machines are produced mainly by vibration, at which they are very good, but their use is unfortunately limited to just this and pressure.

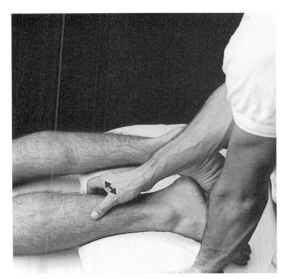

Shaking: using a firm grip from one end of the muscle the whole area can be gently shaken to and fro in a rhythmical way

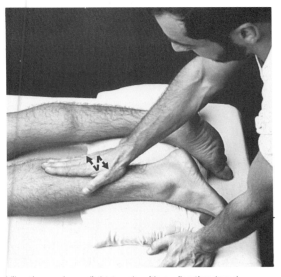

Vibration: using a light touch with a vibrating hand

5
BASIC ROUTINE OF SPORTS MASSAGE

There are as many variations of massage routines as there are therapists. Everyone develops their own style of applying massage through personal experience and instinct. Different therapists using different procedures, which they are competent with, can achieve the same results. To achieve good results it is necessary to have a basic routine, and also it is important to be able to vary this routine according to the needs of the patient.

Most sportsmen require whole body massage. Massage can be given in many different orders. Here are two examples of body massage routines:

1. *Supine*	2. *Prone*
arms	back
chest	shoulders
legs (front)	neck
feet	legs (back)
	feet
Prone	
feet	*Supine*
legs (back)	feet
back	legs (front)
shoulders	chest
neck	arms
	abdomen
Supine	
abdomen	

There are sports where one puts more strain on certain parts of the body; for example, running (legs and back) and canoeing (arms, shoulders, chest, neck, abdomen and back). It is beneficial to concentrate treatment on these parts, and half body massage may be sufficient. It is important that back massage is also included in half body massage – both upper and lower body. The breathing muscles are of central importance in all sports and should be included at regular intervals.

When treating an individual part, for example the front of the leg, one should work in the following order: thigh, shin, foot, shin, thigh. When treating the back of the leg the order should be thigh, calf, foot, calf, thigh. Thus the only correct procedure for deep massage is to work first on the proximal part. This is to improve circulation and clear possible congestion so there is less restriction when starting to work on the distal area. Every part is massaged twice: the first time is mostly diagnostic and to acclimatise the sportsman to the treatment; and the second time is for deeper and more effective massage.

We will use the front thigh as an example:

Begin with long superficial strokes (effleurage) from the knee to the inguinal area covering the front of the leg to spread the oil and acclimatise the patient to the touch. Start the stroke from the distal end and work upwards. This stroking should be returned to several times during the treatment and should be combined with shaking to maintain relaxation.

Kneading (petrissage) techniques may be applied to improve circulation and to soften the muscles. Start these techniques near the inguinal area and proceed towards the knee to improve circulation first in the proximal areas.

Apply deep stroking in a longitudinal direction, gradually working deeper but gently to maintain sensitivity in the finger pads. This is to release tension and to search out problem areas. Again one should start near the inguinal area and work towards the knee treating it in about four or five sections. Although one is first treating from proximal areas, the direction of the strokes is towards the trunk in the direction of venous and lymph flow. It is combined with deep transverse stroking, which is applied particularly to areas where tension is felt. It is easier to identify local trauma and small tense muscle bundles with this technique.

Return to long superficial stroking of the thigh, and then start to massage the shin following the same procedure as above. After that treat the foot and then return to massage the shin again.

Following treatment of the lower leg,

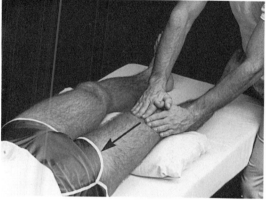

Long superficial strokes applied, starting from the knee towards the inguinal area using both hands

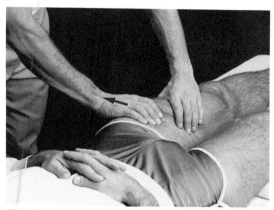

Kneading with both hands working rhythmically, starting from the top of the leg and moving down towards the knee

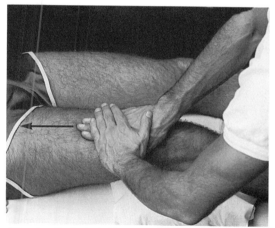

Deep longitudinal stroking applied towards inguinal area using the fingers. Pressure comes mainly from the overlying hand, and movement is made with the arm of the bottom hand

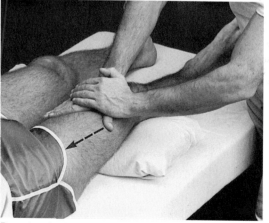

Deep longitudinal stroking applied towards the inguinal area working in sections as one moves down the leg. The thumb is used as a tool under the hand which exerts pressure and movement. This is a most effective technique for applying stretching to local areas

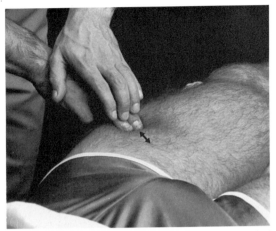

Deep friction applied across the direction of the band of hard muscle, using the fingertips

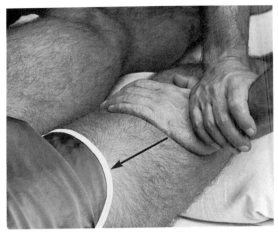

Deep longitudinal stroking applied with the palm reinforced by the other hand

return to the second session on the thigh, which will differ from the first. Start again with superficial strokes, proceeding quickly into kneading and deep strokes. The result of the first treatment is that the muscles are now more relaxed, and it is possible during the second session to use more pressure and to go deeper without causing excessive pain.

Where local scar tissue and/or tight muscle bands were identified previously, deep friction should be used. This should be continued until the scar tissue feels softer and the tightness loosens. This may cause some discomfort and increase tension, so you should then return to superficial stroking techniques to restore relaxation.

Deep stroking and squeezing are used to reach the muscle layers near the bone and will help achieve deeper relaxation and improve circulation.

Finish the massage treatment of a part with superficial stroking and gentle shaking of the muscles.

Whichever part of the body one is treating, the basic massage routine is usually the same:

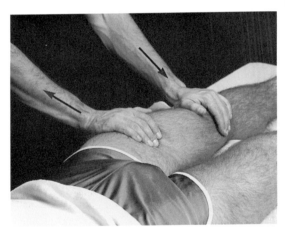

Squeezing, applied by grasping the muscle with both hands and stretching it by pulling with one hand and pushing with the other

Superficial stroking
Kneading
Deep stroking
– longitudinal
– transverse
Superficial stroking

Move on to treat the next area. Then return for the second part of the treatment:

Superficial stroking
Kneading
Deep stroking
Deep friction
Deep stroking
Squeezing
Superficial stroking

There are many other techniques, which can be used for different purposes such as relaxation and stimulation. These can be found in the chapters on general massage techniques and special massage techniques.

In the chapter on specific injury treatment we describe special procedures for treating individual parts of the body with particular regard to sports injuries. The example above shows only the basic approach, which should be followed when treating any part of the body.

With the back the idea of 'proximal' and 'distal' does not have the same significance as it does in the extremities. When treating the back the therapist can work both up the back as well as down. It is good to use both directions as this offers greater versatility in reaching the muscles.

6
ABDOMINAL MASSAGE

Many therapists do not actually include the abdomen in general treatment. This is often due to lack of time or sometimes through insufficient experience in giving it. However, it definitely belongs in a complete treatment. Abdomen massage can be applied in two different ways and it should be often applied using both. More emphasis can be given to one or the other depending on the particular requirements of the sportsman.

When treating excessive tension and strains in the abdomen, massage needs to be directed more specifically in the muscles. Basically the same techniques are used as when treating other parts, but, as there is no support from hard tissue beneath the muscles, small strains and trigger points may flow unnoticed under the hands. Consequently it is necessary for the sportsman to tense the muscles during the treatment so that traumas and tense areas can be found and treated. This can be done simply by getting the sportsman to flex his neck. This tension is also important because tenderness felt in relaxed muscles may be confused with that arising from underlying organs and connective tissues. Traumas most often occur near the attachments of the rectus abdominus muscle to the pubic bone. Muscle tension can be effectively released by treating the lateral border of the rectus abdominus muscle. See the chapter on specific injury treatment.

When abdomen massage forms a part of a general relaxation massage, or when treating bowel dysfunction like constipation and diarrhoea due to general nervous stress and tension, the abdomen should be kept as relaxed as possible. Abdomen massage should always be carried out with the sportsman in the supine position. Some therapists use a sitting position, but this is very awkward and offers no real benefits. The bladder and bowel should be emptied before treatment. To ensure good relaxation the knees should be flexed and the arms should not be above the head, which stretches the abdominal muscles.

Begin treatment by applying gentle superficial stroking from the epigastrium below the base of the sternum down towards the pubic bone, to spread the oil. Massage can then proceed along the course of the large intestine (colon), thus following the direction of intestinal peristalsis. Start just above the right inguinal area and move in a clockwise direction around the abdomen up to the right arcus and then to the epigastrium. Then move across to the left arcus and down to the left inguinal area. Both hands should be used and the fingers should be kept loose to allow them to follow the contours of the abdomen. Superficial stroking is then made in a circular direction and will warm the area and acclimatise the sportsman to having this sensitive area treated. Pressure should be eased slightly as the strokes pass the epigastric area as this is more tender. Pressure should also be eased as the hands move across the lower abdomen to repeat the procedure from the right side again.

Deeper stroking can be applied with the hands working alternately inwards towards the navel with one hand at a time overlapping each other in a constant rhythm. These movements should gradually work their way around the abdomen in a clockwise direction. One should start each cycle above the right inguinal area. This procedure should be repeated at least five times, working more deeply each time. As the pressure is increased the speed of the strokes should be slower, and if pain is caused or muscle tension is felt, pressure should be eased. When sufficient improvement has been achieved one can conclude with superficial stroking in a circular direction along the large intestine.

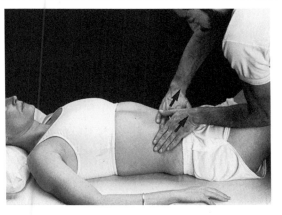

Deep stroking is performed in a clockwise direction starting from the right side of the lower abdomen. Both hands are used alternately. Each stroke starts from the outer part of the abdomen directed towards the navel. As one hand is half way the other hand starts to make another stroke behind it maintaining continual pressure, which should not be released during the treatment. These strokes should gradually work their way round the abdomen, and pressure should be increased with each circuit

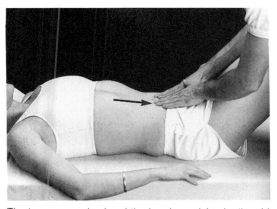

The knees are raised and the hands are lying by the side of the body to relax the abdomen muscles. Both hands are used to apply superficial stroking from the chest directly down towards the pubic bone. The hands should be kept loose to allow them to follow the contours of the abdomen

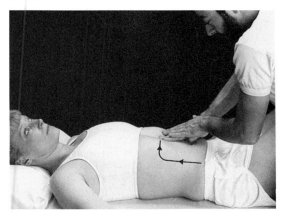

Long strokes applied using the fingers of one hand strengthened by the other hand along the course of the large intestine. Start above the right inguinal ligament, moving around the abdomen to the left side

7
STRETCHING AND MUSCLE ENERGY TECHNIQUE (MET)

Excessive tension may still remain in some muscles after general massage has been completed. This is because the tension has been developing over a very long period, and it may take several massage sessions to normalise the condition. It also usually takes up to two days after treatment for the full effect of the massage to be achieved. Therefore it is necessary to try to restore good function of muscles and joints by using other techniques to reduce this tension so the sportsman can return to normal training without delay and minimise the risk of injury. It is often necessary to work on just a few muscles, or even parts within a muscle, to stretch the tension out and restore muscle balance.

An example of stretching the hamstring muscles. The knee is held straight and the hip joint is gradually flexed. The therapist can use his leg to keep the sportsman's hip and other leg in a fixed position. If the sportsman is allowed to raise the other leg the pelvis will move with the stretched leg and the whole procedure becomes ineffectual. Stretching the hamstrings can also be performed by flexing the hip with the knee bent and then stretching the muscle by gradually extending the knee joint

STRETCHING

This is done as a passive movement and thus one tries to keep the muscle as relaxed as possible. Stretching is done in the opposite direction from the movement made by the action of the muscle, in other words by drawing the muscle attachments away from each other. It is essential to know the location of the attachments, so that it is easy to work out the direction along which the muscles should be stretched.

The movement should be carried out slowly and gently, as any rapid movement will cause a reflex muscle contraction. Proceed to the point where you start to feel resistance and then slowly continue to apply pressure to increase the stretch, but stay within the limits of pain. No tearing or burning sensation should be caused. Move-

An example of stretching the iliotibial tract. The right leg of the sportsman is being adducted to apply the stretch. The therapist is using his right arm against the sportsman's other leg to prevent it from also moving sideways

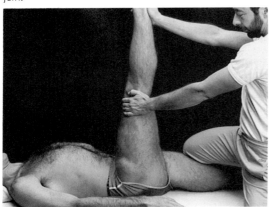

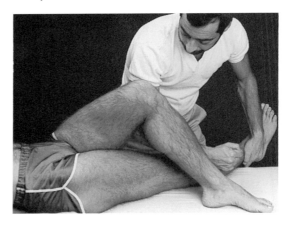

ment may be limited by the joint, where you will feel a hard resistance, or by the muscle, which will be felt as a soft resistance.

These passive stretches should ideally be held for a considerable time (usually about thirty seconds). During this time it should be possible to increase the stretch. Stretching can be repeated after the muscle has been returned to its neutral position and allowed to fully relax (at least five seconds). This relaxation should be enhanced by applying some superficial stroking and shaking to the area being treated. Stretching can be repeated until there is no more progress being made (usually two or three times). To direct a stretch to a particular part of the muscle the therapist can grasp and push the muscle near the area.

In particularly stubborn cases of muscle tension the effect of stretching can be improved by using deep friction on the affected muscle before each stretch.

MUSCLE ENERGY TECHNIQUES (MET)

The main difference to the stretching technique described above is that MET involves the active participation of the sportsman. The muscle energy technique works by creating post isometric relaxation in the muscle, which enables it to be stretched out further. Keeping the muscle relaxed, stretch it out passively as with the previous technique. Stretching should be carried out until increased resistance is felt, and before pain or discomfort are experienced. Holding the part firmly in this position the sportsman should be instructed to contract the muscle using only about twenty per cent of his strength. This contraction is isometric so it is important not to allow any movement. The sportsman should be instructed to contract and relax the muscle slowly and gently to avoid any sudden, jerky movement. The contraction should be held for between five and ten seconds

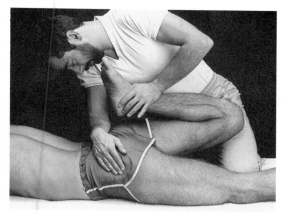

An example of using MET on the quadriceps muscles. The knee is flexed to apply the stretch and the therapist uses his leg to lift the thigh and so apply an initial stretch on the rectus femoris part of the muscle. The arm should press on the back of the hips to stabilise it. The sportsman is asked to push his ankle lightly against the therapist's fixed hand. After ten seconds he is asked to relax fully for a couple of seconds before the therapist slowly pushes down to increase the stretch. Normal flexibility will allow the foot to reach the buttock

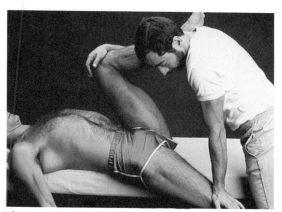

An example of using MET on the iliopsoas muscle. The sportsman lies diagonally on the couch with the leg being treated hanging over the side. The other leg is supported in a flexed position to prevent hip movement. As the hip joint is extended the iliopsoas muscle is pre-stretched. The sportsman is asked to push lightly upwards against the therapist's hand with his knee for ten seconds, and then relax before the stretch is gently increased

depending on the size of the muscle, larger muscles needing more time than smaller ones.

After the contraction the sportsman should be instructed to relax fully. When this has been done the therapist will find that he can draw the part further out without resistance to a new position, thereby increasing the movement. There should only be a delay of a few seconds between the instruction to relax and the movement. This procedure should be repeated until no further progress is being made (usually two to three times).

Where there is tension in a traumatised muscle it may be too painful to use direct MET. Instead, indirect techniques should be used on the antagonist muscle, which should be contracted against resistance in the same way as normal MET for five to ten seconds. This will cause a reflex relaxation effect (reciprocal inhibition) on the traumatised muscle.

Maximal Resisted Contraction (MRC)

It sometimes happens that the sportsman does not respond to this form of gentle MET. In such situations better results may be achieved by the sportsman contracting the muscle maximally for five to ten seconds against a fixed resistance and then taking up the free movement on relaxation. The maximal isometric contraction stretches the muscle in a different way to MET. The belly of the muscle contracts causing a strong stretching to the tendons. As all the muscle fibres are involved in the maximal contraction, the broadening and shortening movement created within the muscle may cause a breakdown of adhesions between fibres.

With passive stretching techniques it is dangerous to cause pain because it may produce muscle or tendon ruptures. With MET and MRC it is safer because, during the active phase, one's own pain reflexes regulate contraction and so prevent excessive stretching.

MRC can also be used in some degree to

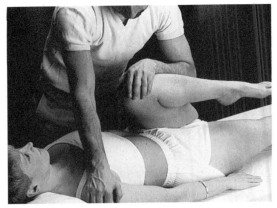

Example of using MRC on the piriformis and other deep buttock muscles. The hip is flexed and the therapist pushes the knee towards the shoulder on the opposite side. A common mistake is to rotate the leg when doing this which causes capsular irritation in the hip joint rather than muscular stretch. The sportsman is asked to push his knee against the therapist's hand, gradually increasing to maximum effort for five to ten seconds and then slowly relaxing. Then the part is stretched further by the therapist. There is no need for lateral rotation of the thigh in this position as this mainly works the adductor muscles and does not help relaxation. The effectiveness of this stretch can be increased by applying compression with the knee, which should be placed midway between the great trochanter and sacral hiatus

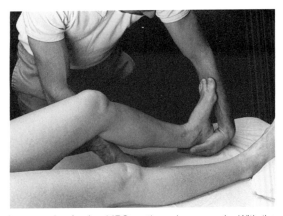

An example of using MRC on the soleus muscle. With the knee in a slightly flexed position to relax the gastrocnemius muscle, the sportsman is asked to push against the therapist's forearm with the top of the foot, gradually building to maximal effort for five to ten seconds and then slowly relaxing. The part is then stretched by pushing the ankle to increase flexion

40

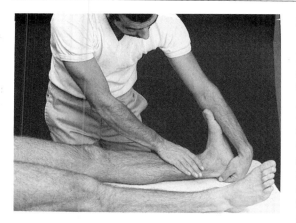

An example of using MRC on the gastrocnemius muscle. To direct the technique to the gastrocnemius muscle, the knee joint should be kept straight. The sportsman is asked to push against the therapist's forearm with the top of the foot, gradually building to maximal effort for five to ten seconds and then slowly relaxing. The part is then stretched by pushing the ankle in flexion

strengthen a muscle and restore its normal function. This is particularly useful where it is not possible to exercise a part, particularly in the case of trauma. Muscle imbalance can be treated in this way as well as with special exercises.

The improved flexibility that results from massage and the other techniques described here can be maintained by instructing the sportsman to carry out exercises which stretch the muscles in the same way as the given techniques. They should be done regularly, at least once a day, and before and after training sessions. It is also important to consider any possible causes of the tension, such as posture, technique, equipment, level and quality of training.

If you use stretching techniques without having given massage first it is important to ensure that the part is warmed up properly before starting to ensure increased elasticity of the soft tissues due to warmth. This can be done with gentle exercise, or by using, for example, heat lamps or heat pads.

8
IDENTIFYING INJURY PROBLEMS

Treating sportsmen with massage can be looked at from two directions. There will be those sportsmen who come to the therapist complaining about a specific problem or fatigue and discomfort, and there will also be those who come for a general massage and are unaware of any particular injury. During massage treatment there will be plenty of time to discuss possible problems.

When the sportsman complains of an injury the first thing to do is to ask questions to try to find out the exact history of the condition. In cases of acute trauma it is essential to discover the direction and nature of the forces involved to know which tissues are likely to be affected. In cases of long-standing injuries the history is even more important because the cause is usually less clear. One should discuss the sportsman's training schedule in some detail to see if there is an overtraining effect with regard to quality or quantity. Other factors such as training environment and equipment can be a matter of importance. It is helpful to know what other treatments the sportsman may have had and what the results were.

The examination begins as soon as the sportsman enters the room. Postural imbalance is often better noticed when the sportsman is not aware of your observation. Muscular tension is noticeable when the person is moving about with rigidity and caution.

In massage, examination and treatment cannot be separated. One should start with gentle massage (superficial and deep stroking) using the very sensitive pads of the fingers to monitor the state of the tissues.

Work systematically and go progressively deeper through the muscle. One should not restrict the treatment just to the muscles; remember the tendons, attachments, ligaments and fascia, which must also be examined and treated.

PATHOLOGICAL CHANGES

Skin: Increased sensitivity, feelings of hot or cold, which can be local to traumatised areas or may be over an area of referred pain (subjective finding). This may be observed by excessive muscle contraction or twitching while being massaged (objective finding).

Numbness and pins and needles occur in areas affected by nerve compression often caused by a tense muscle and fascia. More serious conditions, such as prolapsed disc, can also cause similar symptoms. Constriction in blood supply can also cause similar sensations.

Over traumatised areas there can be localised oedema subcutaneously. This can be noticed by an indentation remaining for a time after sustained pressure with the finger tip.

Over areas of acute trauma and inflammation the skin will appear more red and will have increased temperature.

With long term painful conditions there is usually autonomic nervous system disturbance. The sympathetic system is often overactive, causing constriction of blood vessels. This will be noticed as decreased temperature in the affected areas. There is also sometimes local excessive sweating in the same area.

Subcutaneous layer: Below the skin layer is a variable thickness of fat. This can be felt as a smooth layer or may be soft and nodular. Soft lumps may be felt which are condensed areas of fat. These may be sometimes tender when pressed but are not a source of pain. There may be small lymph nodules, usually in the neck area, appearing when the muscles are particularly tense and may disappear when the muscle becomes relaxed after treatment. These nodules occur naturally and present no danger to the sportsman.

Fascia: The muscles and compartments are lined with fascia which also connects muscle groups and other tissues. Tension in the muscles is often spread to other areas through the fascia, and tenderness will be felt along the path of the connective tissue.

Muscle: Muscle groups, individual muscles, or parts of the muscle can have increased tension or be in spasm. In severe cases this can be even visually observed and is easily felt as hardness. In acute cases this hardness feels smooth on the surface, but with chronic cases it usually appears more wavelike due to the compartmentalised structure of the muscle.

The smallest part of a muscle which may be in contraction is a single motor unit. A few motor units in contraction will feel like a small nodule or piece of string in line with the fibres surrounded by otherwise normal muscle.

Small local ruptures of muscle fibres can be felt as swelling with increased local tension due to pain. Muscle damage will result in restricted joint mobility which can be noticed with passive movement.

Big muscle ruptures can be felt as a hard bulk of contracted muscle which may be some way along the muscle from the actual site of the trauma. The muscle naturally goes into contraction when a break occurs between the attachments. At the site of the trauma a hollow area will be felt if there is not excessive swelling.

Any muscle rupture will result in internal bleeding which will appear as swelling of the muscle, or bruising on the surface which may spread to a very large area.

Any tissue damage will result in the formation of scar tissue, which can be felt as a hard and inflexible area. The formation of scar tissue depends on the size of the trauma and on the individual's ability to form it. Where there is a large formation of scar tissue in a small area it will be felt as a hard lump or knot. Where there is a small amount of scar tissue it may appear as a hollow and stringy feeling in the muscle.

Fibrosis can be felt as a general hardness in a fairly large area along a muscle. It is the result of long-standing contraction in the whole or just part of a muscle. Such areas suffer from a lack of movement, thus restricting normal bloodflow and nutrition. The muscle fibres mat together and lose flexibility which further restricts mobility. Long-standing muscle contraction may be aggravated by micro-traumas which result from repetitive overtraining.

Trigger points are tender spots which appear most commonly in muscle, but may also occur in other tissues. When finding one during massage treatment it will cause radiating pain in surrounding tissue or in a referred area which has been aching. Trigger points will be dealt with in more detail in their own chapter.

Minor muscle atrophies are often difficult to locate by visual inspection and are much more easily identified by palpation. This is not only due to reduced muscle size, but also due to lack of proper tonus.

Tendons: Inflammatory conditions after acute or chronic strains will be noticed as swelling and tenderness along the length of the tendon (tendinitis). In acute cases crepitus, as well as the usual symptoms of inflammation, may be felt inside the tendon sheath as cross friction massage is applied.

Scar tissue and damaged fibres from partially torn tendons will be felt as hard lumps or particles which will be tender in the early stages.

Bursa: These are sacks containing fluid which minimise friction between moving tissues, usually around joints and close to muscle attachments. They are not normally felt, but in cases of acute or chronic strain they may become inflamed. This is felt as a local area of smooth, soft swelling and tenderness. Sometimes this will appear reddened and warm to the touch.

Ligaments: Torn ligaments will cause much inflammation (swelling, heat, pain, redness, bruising) without correct acute treatment. There will be joint instability with marked ligament ruptures. Scar tissue will appear more fibrous, with small hard areas around the injury site.

Ganglion: This is a small hard lump sometimes found on the joint, usually developing after trauma or impact. It is a sack of synovial tissue breaking through the joint capsule. It is often painless, but with excessive use of the joint it may become irritated and tender.

Joints: Even a small amount of swelling in the joint is easy to feel by a change in consistency when massaging areas surrounding the soft tissues.

Restriction of joint movement may be caused by trauma to the joint ligament, capsule, cartilage or bony structures. In these cases a hard resistance is felt which limits the movement. With muscular and tendinous traumas there is a soft resistance, which will yield to some degree when stretched.

Ligament and joint capsule ruptures and fractures cause instability of the joint, but special tests need to be done by a medical practitioner to identify this.

9
SPECIFIC INJURY TREATMENT

This chapter deals with the treatment of specific sports injuries as they relate to massage, by looking at individual muscles and muscle groups throughout the body. Although some diagnostic methods are introduced it is primarily the responsibility of a medical practitioner to diagnose conditions. The main purpose of this chapter is to enable the therapist to understand the conditions and know how best to treat them.

References are made to particular sports where the muscle in question may be more prone to injury. This of course is not intended as a comprehensive list as this would not be possible. It is important also to consider that not all injuries a sports-man may suffer are necessarily 'sports' injuries and may be the result of other activities.

THE LEGS (see illustrations on pp. 54-7).

Quadriceps muscle

The quadriceps femoris consists of four muscles each separated by its own fascias: rectus femoris, vastus lateralis, intermedius and medialis. They form the large muscle group of the front of the thigh. The

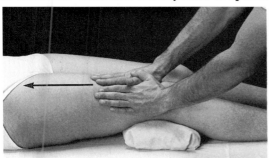

Left: Superficial stroking with flat hands, starting from the knee or foot and running smoothly over the whole area

Deep longitudinal stroking using the thumbs supporting each other. Stretching is applied to a small area of the muscle each time. Deep stroking is started at the proximal area working in sections of a few inches towards the knee. The direction of each stroke is along the muscle fibres towards the inguinal area

Below: Deep longitudinal stroking applied from the origin of the rectus muscle towards the belly of the muscle. The thumb is used merely as a tool with pressure and movement being applied to small areas coming from the overlying hand. Strokes should be short because they are applied in the opposite direction of the return of body fluids. Stroking applied away from the attachment is much more effective than applying it towards the attachment. It is also important to pay attention to the insertion of the quadriceps muscle

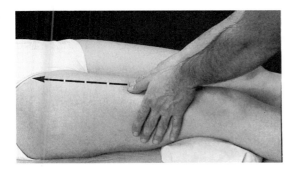

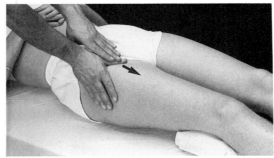

rectus femoris originates in the anterior inferior iliac spine and upper border of the hip joint. The vastus muscles arise from the front surface of the femur. Vastus intermedius covers the articular muscle, which arises in the distal part of the femur and runs into the capsule of the knee joint stretching it. All muscles of the quadriceps connect through the patella ligament and attach on to the tibial tuberosity. Through the patellar retinaculum muscles attach to the medial and lateral condyles of the tibia. The quadriceps extend the knee joint and the rectus part helps with hip flexion.

Strains in these muscles are common in sports requiring explosive power, such as sprinting, jumping, tennis, etc. They occur more often in sportsmen who tend to have excessive external rotation of the shin and in sports where such movements may be forced, like in soccer. It can also occur as a result of inadequate recovery from strength training in many sports, when quick movements are performed. In football and other group games impact trauma is a more common form of injury than overuse. Such injuries can be very deep near the bone, unlike strains which tend to be more superficial. Muscle strains usually occur in the upper part near the origin of the rectus femoris. Overuse problems tend to affect the distal part of the muscle, especially at the insertion of the vastus medialis to the medial side of the shin (tibial tuberosity). Diffuse aching felt in the knee joint is often referred from the quadriceps muscle, tendon and retinaculum as a result of overuse or unsatisfactory recovery from training. Acute strains and trauma to the belly of this big muscle can cause a massive intramuscular bleeding, and effective acute treatment is very important. Massage shoud be applied after two to three days to remove oedema and haematoma and to prevent scar tissue formation. Scar tissue causes pain and dysfunction,

which will prevent the return to normal training. It will also leave the muscle vulnerable to further trauma.

Sartorius muscle

This muscle runs from the anterior superior iliac spine, diagonally and medially down across the front of the thigh, and attaches through the crural fascia on the medial side of the tibial tuberosity. It flexes, abducts, rotates laterally the thigh and flexes and rotates medially the leg. Tension due to overuse appears together with the quadriceps muscle. Deep stroking massage and releasing of the sartorius muscle effectively releases excessive tension in all the muscles in the front of the thigh.

Deep transverse stroking applied on the sartorius muscle running over and across the quadriceps muscle. Longitudinal stroking is not as effective in stretching as the muscle is long and slim. Fingertips reinforced with the other hand are used to stretch the muscle sideways. One should start from the insertion working upwards, because it is far more difficult to find the mid and proximal part otherwise. The knee and hip joints are flexed and the knee is supported on the therapist's hip to bring the sartorius muscle within easy reach

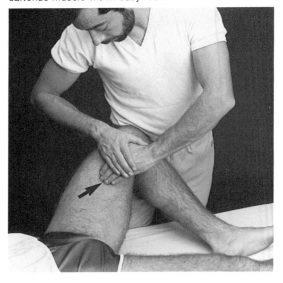

Tensor fascia lata muscle

This muscle arises in the area of the superior iliac spine and extends distal to the greater trochanter attaching to the iliotibial tract. It is a relatively small muscle compared to the other thigh muscles and is often neglected in treatment. It is, however, very important to treat as it often becomes tense and creates further tension in the iliotibial tract. Local pain may be experienced in the front of the hip joint and is often mistaken as a hip joint problem. Pain may also radiate down in front of the thigh. One should remember to treat it routinely when giving leg massage.

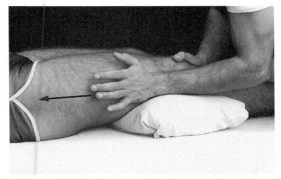

Long strokes applied with the palm of the hand along the iliotibial tract. This should be done with considerable pressure, but slowly to avoid excessive pain

Deep longitudinal stroking applied along the course of the tensor fascia latae muscle with the thumbs supporting each other. This is a small muscle compared to the other thigh muscles. It is treated more comfortably by stroking downwards and not trying to squeeze the muscle against the anterior superior iliac spine by applying massage in an upward direction

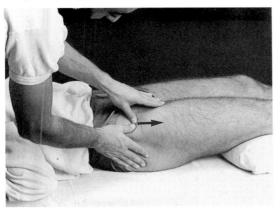

Iliotibial tract

This is a strong tendinous reinforcement of the fascia lata in the lateral aspect of thigh. Fascia lata surrounds all thigh muscles, which have their own fascias separating them from each other. It joins above with the gluteal fascia and runs down to the lateral tibial condyle. Stretching the iliotibial tract releases tension and improves circulation in the whole leg. It is not possible to get good results, when trying to relax the quadriceps muscles, if the tract is not also loosened. Massage is most effective when the main pressure is concentrated between the quadriceps and hamstring muscles.

Adductor group

These form the large group of muscles on the inside of the thigh: adductor longus, magnus and brevis, pectineus and gracilis. They arise in the pubic and ischium bones and attach along the medial and posterior

Strokes along the adductor group should be applied with a large surface like the flat of the hand as this area is usually tender. These muscles can be reached more easily when the leg is held in a flexed, abducted and outwardly rotated position. The leg will remain relaxed as the knee is rested on a pillow or the therapist's hip

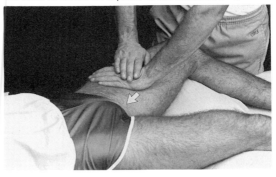

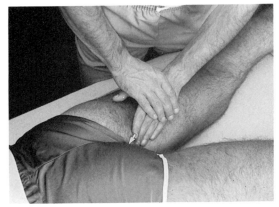

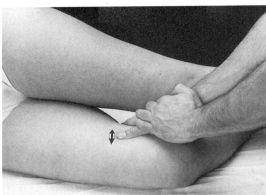

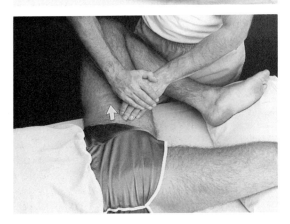

Top: Longitudinal strokes applied with a flat hand. Deeper effect is acquired by using the fingertips more and reinforcing the pressure with the other hand. In the supine position the muscle origins in the ischial tuberosity are much easier to reach

Middle: When treating specific injuries a good position to use is lying on the side being treated, with the leg slightly bent at the hip and knee. Deep friction is applied with the thumb reinforced with the other hand

Below: Deep longitudinal strokes applied with the fingers, reinforced with the other hand, near the origin of the adductor muscles. Strokes should be short as they are applied down the leg in the opposite direction to the returning circulation. Deep stroking towards the belly of the muscle from the attachment creates a good stretching effect on the origin in the pubic bone

side of the femur from the lesser trochanter to the medial epicondyle. The gracilis muscle attaches with the sartorius muscle on the medial aspect of the tibial tuberosity.

The most vulnerable of these muscles to sports injury is the adductor longus, which is often strained when the leg is outwardly rotated and abducted simultaneously, for example when drawing back the leg after kicking backwards in skating and skiing, after jumping or crossing fences in hurdling, and when kicking a football with the inside of the foot. Trauma is most often located near its attachment on the pubic bone. There may also be extreme tenderness and pain at the attachment of the rectus abdominus muscle in the same area due to connections between fascias. Excessive tension may develop in breast stroke swimmers and can become chronic, usually affecting the attachment at the inside of the knee. Trauma in the adductor attachment has a tendency to turn into a chronic painful condition, and so after the initial acute treatment it is very important to apply deep cross friction massage to prevent fibrosis and the formation of scar tissue and to improve circulation. Strains towards the belly of the muscles may be more painful, but they respond well to massage treatment and heal quickly.

Anterior compartment

This comprises the muscles of the extensor group of the leg: tibialis anterior, extensor digitorum longus and extensor hallucis longus. The muscles attach to the lateral surface of the tibia, interosseus membrane and fibula running down to the foot. They dorsiflex and turn the foot inwards.

Pain in the front of the shin may be caused by direct impact trauma, which is common in sports like football, resulting in inflammation and bleeding. This may cause increased pressure in the muscle group which is surrounded by tight fascia (anterior compartment syndrome). This condition can become so severe that circulation becomes totally blocked if training is not stopped in time. In a few cases even acute surgery has been needed, because long-standing ischemia inevitably leads to muscle necrosis. To prevent this, effective acute treatment: rest, ice, compression and elevation (RICE) is essential, and massage is contraindicated in such acute conditions.

Anterior compartment syndrome due to overuse can appear quite suddenly, and pain increases with running or walking until it becomes impossible to continue. This condition is most often found in runners, but it can also occur in racket sports like tennis and squash as a result of strain due to playing on a hard surface. It also occurs in cycling from hard pulling on the pedals. The build-up of tension in this area often goes unnoticed or is ignored by the sportsman until an acute onset of the pain. Exceptionally high effort for which he has not prepared or trained for may also be a causative factor. Acute treatment is essential in the early stage to reduce the intrafascial pressure and pain which will make massage treatment impossible. The problem can become chronic if either the post acute treatment has not been sufficient or if the symptoms are only minor so the sportsman is able to ignore them. It can be relieved and may even completely disappear with rest and anti-inflammatory drugs, only to recur as soon as training begins to increase again. Regular deep stroking massage during training has proved to be a very effective preventative measure as it improves circulation, reduces muscle tension and stretches fascia, thus reducing intrafascial pressure.

Tibialis anterior is the largest muscle in the shin. Inflammation can occur in the tendon sheath (tibialis anterior syndrome) and is usually due to acute overuse like interval sprint training, football, squash and other racket sports. Activities involving strong dorsiflexion of the foot like hill running and cross country running can also cause this condition. Inflammation of the tendon sheath can arise in the front of the ankle as a result of over-tightened or badly fitting shoes. In acute cases crepitation may be felt when giving deep friction massage in a transverse direction to the tendon. In addition to this technique, deep stroking massage should be applied to the muscle to release tension pulling on the tendon.

Peroneus muscles

The peroneus longus muscle originates from the proximal part of the fibula and tibiofibular joint. The peroneal brevis is a shorter muscle which originates from the mid-third of the lateral surface of the fibula. The peroneus tertius is a slip of muscle from the long extensor muscle of the toes. There are rare cases of a fourth peroneal muscle arising from the lateral surface of the fibula. Tendons of all these muscles run behind and under the lateral malleolus to the tarsal and metatarsal bones. They pronate and plantar flex the foot.

The peroneal muscles are surrounded by

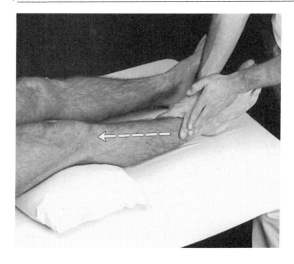

Top: Deep longitudinal stroke applied with the thumb along the muscles of the shin. The area should be treated with slow strokes in small sections

Middle: Deep transverse stroking with the fingertips reinforced with the other hand to separate the anterior tibial muscle and the long extensor muscle of toes from the tibial bone

Below: Deep longitudinal stroking with the thumb, away from the origin of the muscles of the anterior compartment. This should be done as a short stroke as it is in the opposite direction of the venous and lymphatic flow

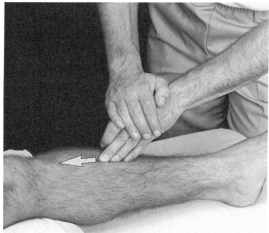

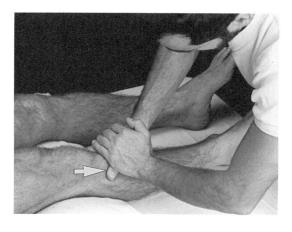

their own fascia (lateral compartment). Painful conditions appear mainly with acute strain and chronic overuse when the sportsman has a stepping fault: the foot has a tendency to rotate inwards during the power phase. Pain may be felt near the knee and often radiates to the lateral side of the foot. Stroking techniques can effectively be applied, and special attention should be given to treatment of the proximal area.

Gluteal muscles (maximus, medius and minimus)

This muscle group originates along the lateral border of the sacrum, sacrotuberous ligament, the ilium and iliac crest. The medius and minimus attach to the greater trochanter of the femur. The gluteus maximus attaches to the gluteal tuberosity on the back of the femur and the iliotibial tract, effecting tension in the thigh and function of the knee. The main function of the gluteal muscles is to extend the hip joint and raise the trunk from a forward bending position. They are therefore the main muscles involved in lifting. All gluteal muscles abduct the femur, but the maximus can also adduct due to its attachment to the gluteal tuberosity. The medius and minimus can also flex the hip joint, abduct, rotate it both laterally and medially depending on which part of the muscle is contracting. This muscle group is

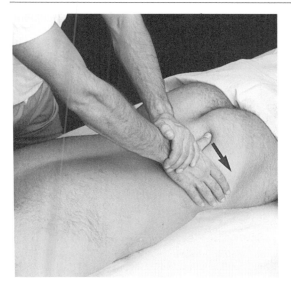

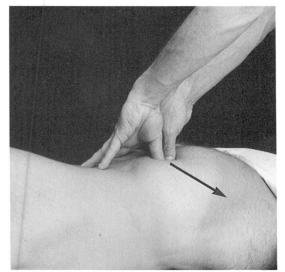

Above: Deep transverse stroking with the thumb along the iliac creast, at the origin of the gluteus maximus

Above right: Deep longitudinal stroking with the thumbs supporting each other. Strokes are performed in the direction of the course of muscle fibres from the sacrum and origin of the gluteus maximus muscle

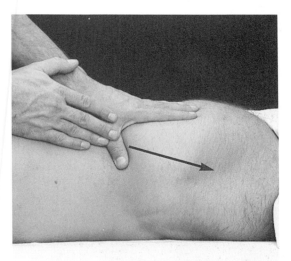

Deep longitudinal stroking along the course of the gluteus muscle applied by the thumb, reinforced with the other hand. Strokes should be performed fairly slowly to avoid irritation and the tensing up of the muscles

very important in maintaining an upright posture in all activities.

The front thigh muscles are often believed to be the most important muscle group in many sporting activities. In sports which entail a large effort with the legs, like running, jumping, weight lifting, rowing and so on, it is in fact the gluteals which are the major working muscles. In leg massage these should never be neglected. Most injuries are concentrated around the distal attachments as the muscular part is very strong. Overuse injuries tend to occur in sports which require repetitive effort with the legs in a relatively high position, like in cross country running, orienteering and climbing. In sports involving repetitive effort with a relatively limited range of movement, as in endurance running and walking, fibrosis and scar tissue tend to build up along the origin of the gluteus maximus over the sacroiliac joint. Minor problems in these muscles may not result in pain locally but may cause tension to build up in the hamstrings. Deep stroking massage along the inferior border of the superior iliac crest and lateral borders of the sacrum and coccyx is very effective treatment. The attachments around the hip joint are very deep and are therefore difficult to reach, but if the muscles are sufficiently relaxed it is possible to effectively treat them.

Top: Small to and fro movements applied with the fingertips reinforced with the other hand to create pressure in the deep gluteal muscles and to induce relaxation

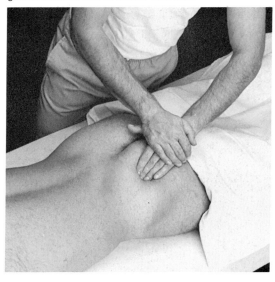

Below: Longitudinal stroking applied with the elbow along the gluteal muscles to reach deep in this big muscle group. This may be useful when the muscles are so tense that it is difficult to apply hand stroking techniques

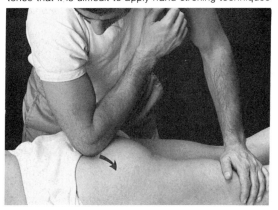

Piriformis muscle

Pain radiating from the buttocks and travelling down the leg (sciatica) can be caused by tension in the piriformis muscle. Its origin is at the sacrum; it lies very deep in the buttocks and attaches to the greater trochanter. The piriformis laterally rotates, abducts and extends the femur. The sciatic nerve passes under the piriformis or sometimes even through it.

Muscle tension can cause nerve entrapment. Acupuncture or injection of local anaesthetic is often the most effective treatment, because the muscle is located deeply and is difficult to reach with massage. Good results can sometimes be achieved by combining stretching with strong sharp pressure over the muscle.

Iliotibial tract

The iliotibial tract should be treated thoroughly when releasing tension in the hamstring muscles. It is an important structure for lateral stability of the knee. The joint capsule can be felt between it and the lateral collateral ligament. The iliotibial tract is free to move back and forth across the lateral side of the epicondyle when the knee is flexed and extended. Tendinous inflammation can develop here if there is excessive tension along the tract. Pain in the lateral side of the knee is common in sports which involve a lot of running (runner's knee). The onset of pain is usually felt after running for some distance, and it then becomes progressively worse until it is impossible to continue. Running downhill increases the pain, and runners with excessive pronation are at greater risk. In addition to tendinitis there may also be bursitis and even swelling of the knee joint. Excessive tension along the tract disturbs normal rotation in the joint causing capsular stretch. Bursitis should not be treated by massage but longitudinal stroking massage over the iliotibial tract

Top: Longitudinal stroking using the elbow to stretch the iliotibial tract. This is a very powerful technique and it should be done slowly. It is often easier to perform if applied in a few sections

Middle: Deep stroking using the thumb reinforced with the other hand at the beginning of the iliotibial tract and at the insertion of the gluteus maximus muscle. By moving upwards the therapist reaches the attachment of the piriformis muscle which is commonly painful with lower back troubles

Below: Deep stroking applied with the thumb starting from the insertion of the biceps muscle of the thigh and iliotibial tract

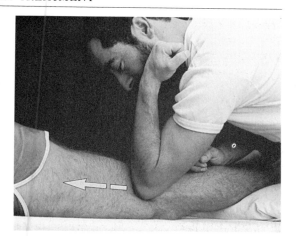

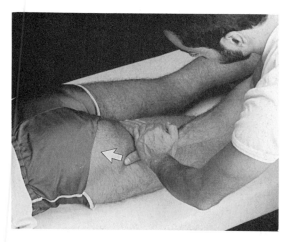

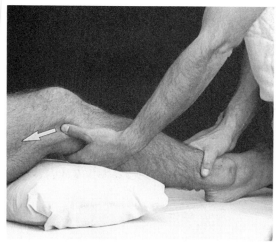

can be applied to relieve the condition. Local tension can often be found at the tenomuscular junction located just below the greater trochanter, and deep transverse stroking can be effectively applied. Stretching should also be done.

Hamstring muscles

This group consists of three muscles: semitendinosus, semimembranosus, and biceps femoris. They extend the hip joint working effectively in lifting and flexing the knee joint in activities like running. The biceps femoris is the only lateral rotator of the leg, and the semitendinosus and membranosus work in the opposite directions. The semitendinosus muscle has its origin in the ischial tuberosity and inserts into the medial tibial condyle. The semimembranosus runs similarly, and part of it forms the oblique popliteal ligament. It is thus even more closely related to medial stability of the knee, and tension along it should be considered in painful disorders on the medial side of the knee joint. The biceps femoris also has its origins in the ischial tuberosity and insert into the lateral aspect of the tibia and fibula. It is an important structure in the lateral stability of the knee joint. When treating knee pain by releasing tension in the iliotibial tract one should also apply deep longitudinal stroking to the biceps femoris muscle.

Superficial muscles

Bones

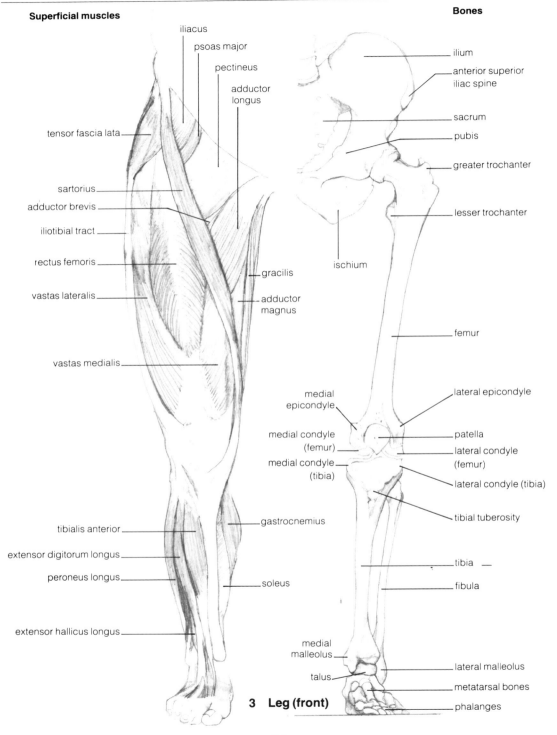

iliacus

psoas major

pectineus

adductor longus

tensor fascia lata

sartorius

adductor brevis

iliotibial tract

rectus femoris

vastas lateralis

gracilis

adductor magnus

vastas medialis

ilium

anterior superior iliac spine

sacrum

pubis

greater trochanter

lesser trochanter

ischium

femur

medial epicondyle

medial condyle (femur)

medial condyle (tibia)

lateral epicondyle

patella

lateral condyle (femur)

lateral condyle (tibia)

tibial tuberosity

tibialis anterior

extensor digitorum longus

peroneus longus

extensor hallicus longus

gastrocnemius

soleus

tibia

fibula

medial malleolus

talus

lateral malleolus

metatarsal bones

phalanges

3 Leg (front)

Deep muscles

Bones

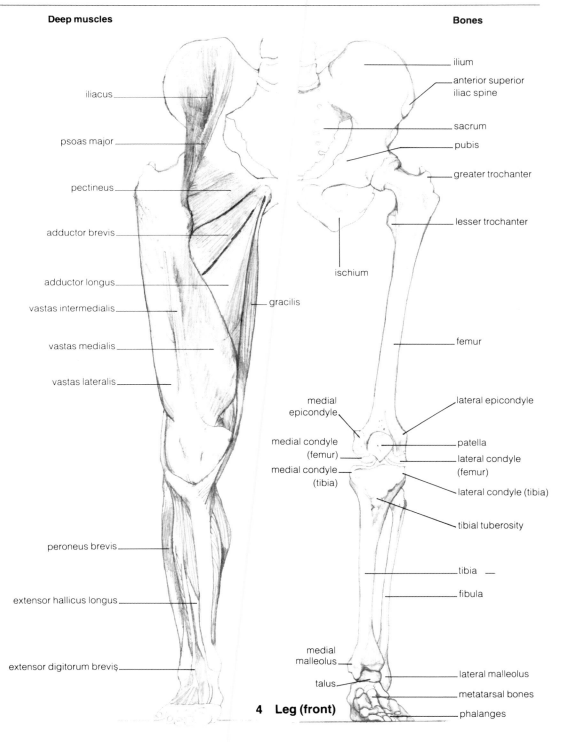

iliacus

psoas major

pectineus

adductor brevis

adductor longus

vastas intermedialis

vastas medialis

vastas lateralis

gracilis

ilium

anterior superior
iliac spine

sacrum

pubis

greater trochanter

lesser trochanter

ischium

femur

medial
epicondyle

medial condyle
(femur)

medial condyle
(tibia)

lateral epicondyle

patella

lateral condyle
(femur)

lateral condyle (tibia)

tibial tuberosity

peroneus brevis

extensor hallicus longus

extensor digitorum brevis

tibia

fibula

medial
malleolus

talus

lateral malleolus

metatarsal bones

phalanges

4   Leg (front)

55

Superficial muscles

Bones

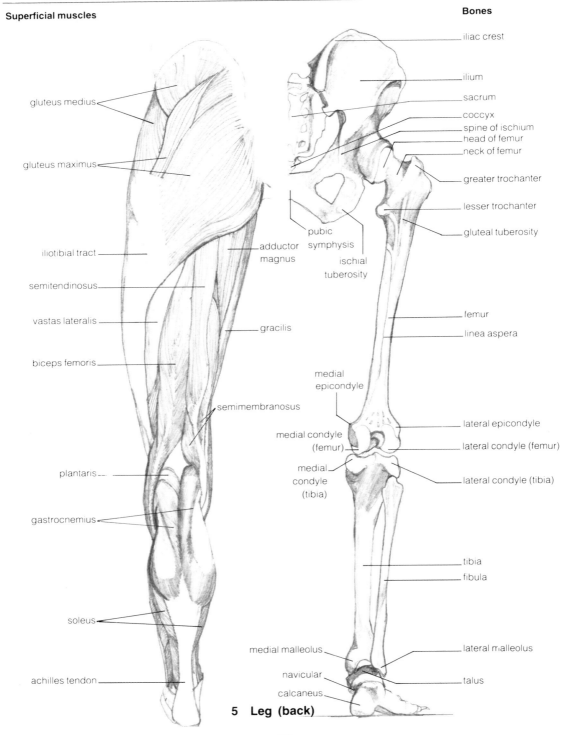

gluteus medius

gluteus maximus

iliotibial tract

semitendinosus

vastas lateralis

biceps femoris

semimembranosus

plantaris

gastrocnemius

soleus

achilles tendon

adductor
magnus

gracilis

pubic
symphysis

ischial
tuberosity

medial
epicondyle

medial condyle
(femur)

medial
condyle
(tibia)

medial malleolus

navicular

calcaneus

iliac crest

ilium

sacrum

coccyx

spine of ischium

head of femur

neck of femur

greater trochanter

lesser trochanter

gluteal tuberosity

femur

linea aspera

lateral epicondyle

lateral condyle (femur)

lateral condyle (tibia)

tibia

fibula

lateral malleolus

talus

5 Leg (back)

56

Deep muscles

Bones

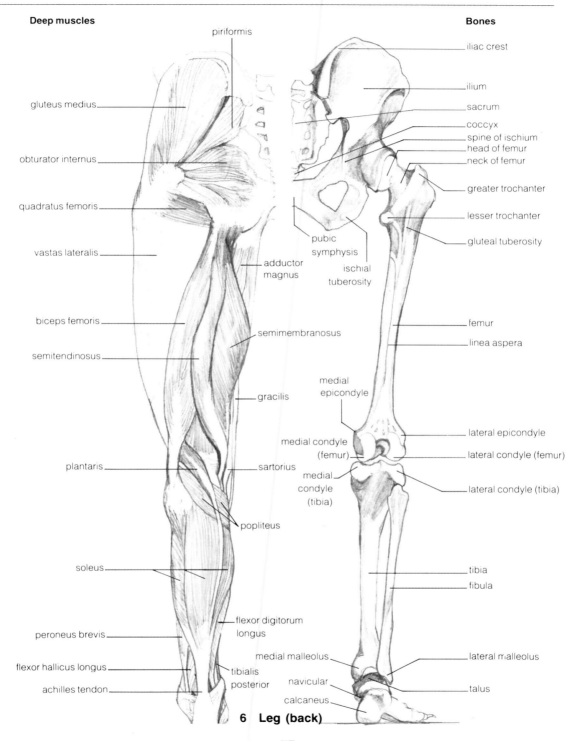

piriformis

gluteus medius

obturator internus

quadratus femoris

vastas lateralis

biceps femoris

semitendinosus

plantaris

soleus

peroneus brevis

flexor hallicus longus

achilles tendon

adductor magnus

semimembranosus

gracilis

sartorius

popliteus

flexor digitorum longus

tibialis posterior

pubic symphysis

ischial tuberosity

medial epicondyle

medial condyle (femur)

medial condyle (tibia)

medial malleolus

navicular

calcaneus

iliac crest

ilium

sacrum

coccyx

spine of ischium

head of femur

neck of femur

greater trochanter

lesser trochanter

gluteal tuberosity

femur

linea aspera

lateral epicondyle

lateral condyle (femur)

lateral condyle (tibia)

tibia

fibula

lateral malleolus

talus

6 Leg (back)

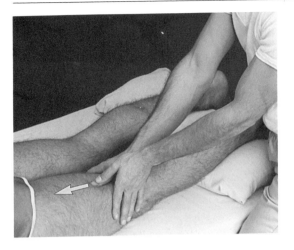

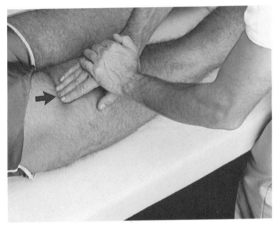

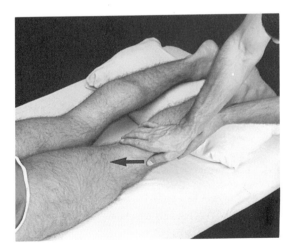

Top: Stroking with one thumb pressing on the other to reach deeply between the hamstring muscles to separate them and stretch the fascia

Middle: Applying stroking with the fingers supported by the other hand to reach deeply to induce a stretch away from the attachments of the hamstring muscles at the ischial tuberosity. Strokes should be very short as they are applied towards the belly of the muscle, against the venous and lymphatic flow

Below: Short longitudinal strokes with the thumb applied to the biceps femoris muscle starting from the tendon

Strains in the hamstring muscles are common to sports which involve quick, powerful flexion of the knee like sprinting and middle distance running, jumping, soccer and racket sports. Intramuscular bleeding can occur, and acute treatment is very important to prevent this. Vulnerability increases if the sportsman neglects the hamstrings in training by paying more attention to the front thigh muscles. After acute symptoms have subsided massage is essential to remove scar tissue and improve circulation which would otherwise cause complications when training is resumed. Chronic and overuse condition tend to occur near the muscle origins along the ischial tuberosity and are more common among sprinters. Scar tissue and localised tension can normally be felt quite easily on palpation, and deep friction massage is effective treatment.

Traumatic back pain such as prolapsed disc, facet joint dysfunction and ligament problems, may all result in both local back pain and radiated pain to the legs (ischias). These cause muscle tension in all muscles in the back of the leg. With prolapsed disc problems it sometimes occurs that there are no back symptoms at all, and moving the back may also be completely pain free. The only symptom may be that the hamstring muscles go into spasm to protect the nerve root from being pulled and damaged by the prolapsed disc. Straight leg raising is limited on one side and no forceful stretching should be made. When treating hamstring problems which have not been caused by any obvious leg effort then the lower back should be considered. Lower back dysfunction may even cause chronic knee aches due to muscle and fascia tension.

Popliteus muscle

This muscle run downwards and diagonally across the back of the knee. It goes from the lateral femoral condyle to the posteromedial surface of the tibia and also inserting into the posterior portion of the lateral meniscus. Dynamically it stabilises the lateral side of the knee and draws the lateral meniscus backwards when the knee is bent.

Excessive tension can cause pain in or behind the knee which may only be felt during movement or when loading the joint in the flexed position. This is often cured by a single joint manipulation. Pain may return after a while if the popliteal

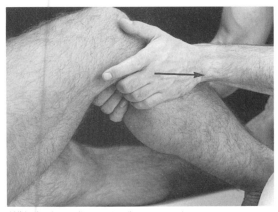

With the knee flexed the fingers can be used to penetrate deeply into the popliteal area and apply deep transverse stroking and stretching sideways and downwards

muscle and the iliotibial system, which also affect lateral stability of the knee, are not also massaged and stretched properly. Tension is seldom isolated to just this muscle. There is usually combined muscle tension causing imbalance in the rotation of the lower leg in relation to the upper part. Normal walking and running involves a smooth external rotation when the leg moves backwards, and internal rotation on forward movement.

Plantaris muscle

This is a delicate muscle which has its origin at the lateral femoral condyle with the gastrocnemius. It forms into a long tendon which passes medially between the soleus and gastrocnemius muscles and attaches to the medial side of the calcaneal tendon.

Functionally the plantaris muscle is not notable, but tension can develop in it causing pain and sometimes even swelling in the back of the knee. Tightness in the long tendon can cause irritation at the inferior medial aspect of the gastrocnemius. Deep friction is effective treatment, especially when applied at an early stage, across the tendon and muscle.

Longitudinal stroking applied with the fingers reinforced with the other hand to the popliteus and plantaris muscles. The direction of the strokes is towards the thigh following the course of the muscle fibres. In the back of the knee lymphatic nodules are sometimes felt: these should be avoided to prevent irritation

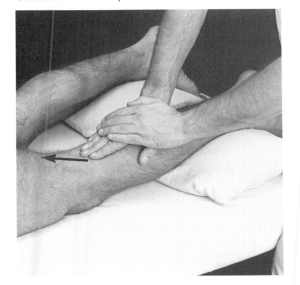

Posterior superficial compartment

Gastrocnemius muscle: The two heads of the gastrocnemius muscle attach to the medial and lateral femoral condyles. The lateral head merges with the posterior knee capsule stabilising the knee in this direction. This is important in movements where the knee is flexed and the capsule cannot give stability. It inserts into the calcaneal tendon (Achilles tendon). The gastrocnemius extends the ankle and flexes the knee.

Muscle strain often occurs in sports which involve quick movements on hard surfaces, like volleyball, badminton and other racket sports, and wherever hard running is required. Tension can develop in the muscle in sports like cycling where it works mostly isometrically. Excessive tension in the calf muscles can cause pain in the back of the knee and can be effectively treated by massage. Tension makes the muscle more vulnerable to trauma, which usually affects the medial musculotendinous junction. Massage should start after two to three days to prevent scar tissue formation and to speed up recovery. Untreated injuries often lead to chronic painful conditions and can cause repeated trauma. Overuse injuries of the gastrocnemius are common to sports which involve running on hard surfaces, and are mainly due to microtrauma. The lateral side is usually affected most and may relate to worn or badly fitting shoes, or excessive pronation. Massage using deep strokes and friction works well in restoring normal muscle function. To prevent this condition regular massage and stretching are essential.

The soleus muscle: This originates at the proximal ends of the fibula and tibia and attaches through the Achilles tendon into the calcaneum. It is primarily a plantarflexor of the ankle joint; as it attaches below the knee joint this is not affected. It can sustain injury through similar conditions as the gastrocnemius. Growth of the soleus muscle due to effective training may lead to posterior compartment syndrome. Symptoms usually appear after harder training sessions when there is increased tension and production of metabolic products like lactic acid. The medial side of the muscle is most often affected, and painful conditions often appear with deep compartment syndrome. There may also be pain at the medioposterior border of the tibia because of irritation of the fascia. This condition can become chronic in people who have stepping faults (excessive pronation), flat foot and tendency to valgus in the ankle joint. These conditions can be treated effectively by deep stroking and friction massage.

Posterior deep compartment

This contains the following muscles: tibialis posterior, flexor hallicus longus and digitorum longus. These muscles arise from the upper parts of the tibia, fibula and interosseus membrane. They have long tendons, which go around the medial malleolus, attaching to the bones on the

Superficial longitudinal stroking of the gastrocnemius and soleus muscles, using both hands working side by side from the heel to the back of the thigh

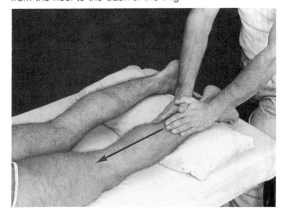

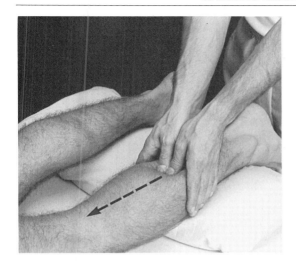

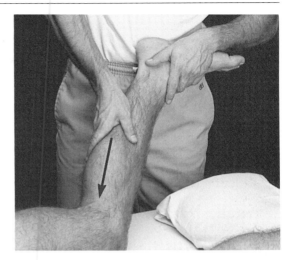

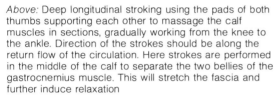

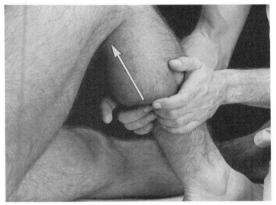

Above: Deep longitudinal stroking using the pads of both thumbs supporting each other to massage the calf muscles in sections, gradually working from the knee to the ankle. Direction of the strokes should be along the return flow of the circulation. Here strokes are performed in the middle of the calf to separate the two bellies of the gastrocnemius muscle. This will stretch the fascia and further induce relaxation

Above right: The lower leg is held in an elevated position to achieve better relaxation on the gastrocnemius muscles and also as a comfortable position for the therapist. The thumb and fingers apply deep stroking to the calf

Middle right: The foot is fixed under the therapist's leg to hold the knee and the ankle in flexion to ensure relaxation of the calf muscles. Deep stroking is performed with the fingertips of both hands along the calf muscles, working towards the back of the knee joint

Below right: The foot is hooked over the other leg to flex the knee and relax the calf muscle. Short deep transverse strokes are applied on the lateral side with the thumb, using the fingers for anchorage. Muscles and fascia are stretched away from the posterior border of the tibial bone

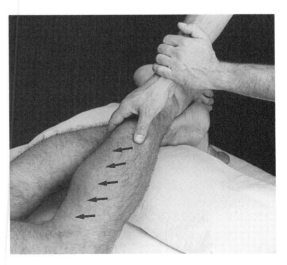

plantar side of the foot. They play a major part in all movement and stability of the ankle joint and cause plantar flexion and supination of the foot.

Painful conditions can develop in these muscles in all sports involving heavy repetitive leg work on hard surfaces and particularly long distance running. The basic cause of the problem may be a stepping problem (supination or pronation

61

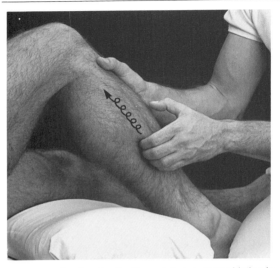

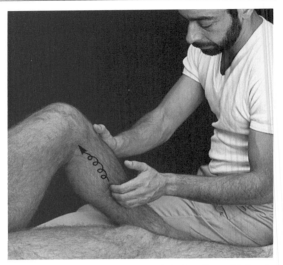

The foot is fixed under the therapist's leg. Deep friction is applied on the lateral border of the tibia to induce stretching of the muscles and fascia away from the bone. This achieves relaxation of the muscles and reduces pressure in the posterior compartments of the calf

The foot is fixed under the therapist's leg. Deep friction is applied on the medial border of the tibia. This is the main treatment method for 'shin splints'. The therapist's aim is to break adhesions which often form with long-standing strain

of the foot), anatomical features like a low foot arch and valgus or varus of the ankle. Depending on the anatomical structure of the foot and stepping style, pain can appear on the lateral, or more commonly the medial, side of tibial bone.

Medial tibial stress syndrome, more commonly called 'shin splints', results in pain at varying heights along the medial side of the shin, but most commonly symptoms appear between the lower and the middle third. This pain can arise due to many reasons. Muscles can build up through training, but the fascia surrounding them may not be able to accommodate them. Increased pressure in the posterior compartment results from long-standing muscle tension and swelling due to inadequate recovery. It may develop suddenly due to acute swelling and local irritation after impact trauma or acute overuse. Without effective treatment the condition tends to become chronic and difficult to manage. The medioposterior border of the tibia may be very tender when palpated

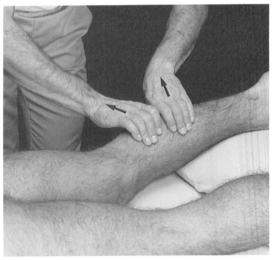

Squeezing of the calf muscles by taking a firm grip from the belly of the muscle and pulling and pushing it sideways. This causes an effective shearing between the muscles and bone

due to periosteal inflammation, and soft resistance can often be felt due to swelling of connective tissue. Anti-inflammatory drugs and rest often give relief, only for the symptoms to return when training is resumed. In operative treatment the fascia of the posterior compartment is divided medially to release pressure.

Massage treatment should be applied with deep friction from the medial border of the tibia backwards to remove adhesions, which tend to form along the bone in chronic cases, and to stretch fascia. Deep longitudinal strokes release muscle tension and so also reduce pressure in both deep and superficial posterior compartments, as both are always simultaneously involved. Tenderness in the medial borders of the soleus and gastrocnemius gradually disappears with massage.

Except in really acute conditions there is seldom need for complete rest. Massage treatment should be applied daily, and most days this can be done by the sportsman giving himself local self massage according to the advice of the therapist. Massage has proved to be effective even in some cases where surgery has failed. If there is no response to treatment after two weeks of effectively applied treatment, this may be due to severe periostitis, myositis ossificans or stress fracture. Medical advice should thus be sought in these cases.

Achilles tendon

Local hardness with pain and tenderness can appear in the middle of the tendon and is usually associated with severe calf pain following intensive exercise or sudden stress. This means there is a partial rupture of the tendon. Total rupture can occur when a sudden extreme load is put through the calf muscle, and is more common in tennis and sports played on hard surfaces and sprinters pushing off too hard at the start. This condition requires surgical repair. With minor ruptures, deep friction massage is sufficient treatment to prevent scar tissue formation (four to five days after trauma). If a large lump of scar tissue has already formed it should be removed by operation, not by massage.

Long-standing strain on hard surfaces, as in long distance running, and tension in the calf muscles may lead to Achilles tendinitis. The inflammation causes pain and swelling. In acute cases crepitus may be felt when the skin is moved over the underlying tissues. Friction massage is beneficial and should be applied to reduce swelling, improve circulation and to break adhesions. Effective treatment is vital to prevent it developing into a long term chronic condition.

Some long distance runners suffer Achilles tendinitis caused by high heel tabs on their shoes. Tenderness and pain with a thickening of the tendon is usually found one inch above the point where the heel tab makes contact with the tendon. Frictional massage and advice to change shoes or cut away the heel tab is effective.

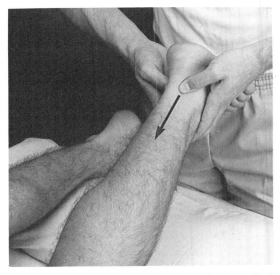

With the lower leg held in an elevated position and with the front of the ankle cradled in the fingers and the sole supported by the therapist, the tips and pads of the thumbs apply stroking along sides of the Achilles tendon

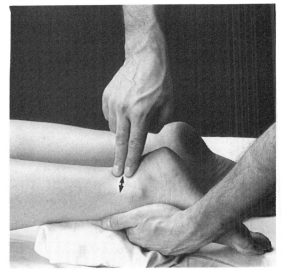

Ligaments and tendons

Ligament sprains to the ankle are common both in sport and everyday life, and are caused by sudden forced lateral movement of the ankle. After the acute phase of partial ligament ruptures it is important to apply deep friction massage. This prevents the formation of scar tissue and adhesions, which are inelastic and can restrict movement. They prevent the growth of new more tolerable fibrous tissues which need to replace those damaged, and so treatment helps in the regeneration process. Massage treatment should start after four to five days with deep friction. Stroking techniques should be used if there is swelling to be removed. Active movements should be performed as soon as possible, and weightbearing allowed if there is not excessive swelling. More serious ruptures require an operation, and thus examination by a medical practitioner is essential.

There are several long tendons running beside the ankle, and with inflammation, massage treatment is the same as with

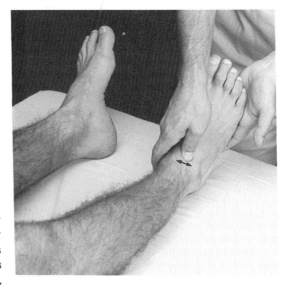

Deep friction to the extensor tendons of the ankle. In tendinitis, strokes should be applied with a to and fro movement across the tendon, not along the course of it as this is the movement which causes the condition

tendinitis and tenosynovitis, usually gentle deep friction directed across the course of the tendons.

Massage can be used similarly for treating all other joints. To avoid unnecessary repetition only the ankle joint is shown as an example.

The foot

Massage of the foot is good for promoting general relaxation. The foot carries the heaviest burden of the body and many overuse conditions are common to it. Massage and stretching promote circulation and help recovery. The plantar aponeurosis runs from the calcaneus to the tendon of the short toe flexors and toe ligaments. It can become strained in sports involving vigorous take-off and landing on hard surfaces. It may become inflamed (plantar fascitis) due to long-standing repetitive strain and tension. Excessive pronation of the foot and shoes with

Deep friction to the lateral ankle ligaments to break adhesions and scar tissue

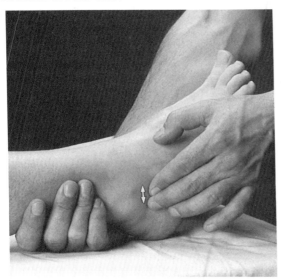

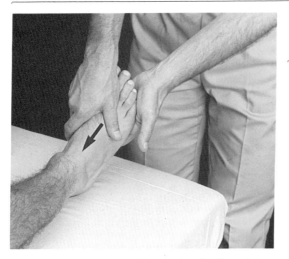

With the sole of the foot resting against the therapist's hand, the fingers and thumb of the other hand apply superficial stroking to the dorsal surface of the foot. This is mainly to stretch the fascia

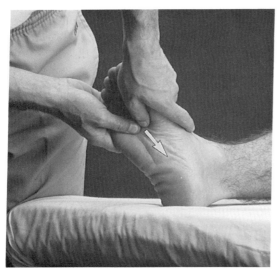

The pads of the thumbs supporting each other to achieve more effective pressure in deep stroking techniques to the muscles in the sole of the foot. Direction of strokes is towards the heel

insufficient arch support can make the sportsman more vulnerable to this overuse injury. Friction massage is useful treatment in releasing a tense aponeurosis and will improve circulation and promote recovery. It should not be applied near the calcaneus attachment – because of the thickness of the soft tissue it would be necessary to use so much pressure that it would merely irritate the junction between bone and tendon.

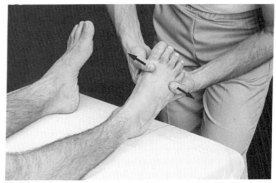

The foot is grasped from both sides, pressing the fingers into the mid sole and stretching with thumbs across the metatarsal area

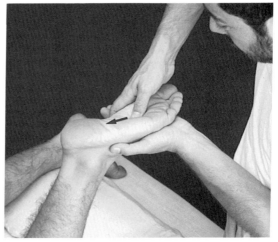

Prone: alternative approach to massage the feet. The foot can be easily lifted to an appropriate height for treatment. In this position only one hand can be used for treatment as the other hand is used to support the leg

THE BACK (see illustrations on pp. 78–9).

The spine is the most complex mechanical structure of the body consisting of twenty-five weightbearing structures (vertebrae and the sacrum). There are twenty-three discs allowing movement and absorbing shock between each vertebra and accounting for one-third of the height of the whole column. There are two synovial joints between each vertebra, and numerous ligaments, tendons and muscles which bind them all together. With so many moving structures involved, the back is particularly vulnerable to injury.

Nearly everybody has had back pain at some time in their life and many suffer long-standing problems. Sportsmen are no exception, and are in fact more at risk due to the greater stresses they place on their bodies. The most common sports for back injuries are weight-lifting, rugby, butterfly swimming and sports where one side of the body is more dominant, like throwing sports, most ball sports and racket sports. The back muscles are also at risk in sports which involve quick movements with rotation and bending the spine, which can become strained if coordination of the movement fails for some reason. If training is performed predominantly on one side it can create a functional curvature of the spine to the same side. This can become a permanent scoliosis in the long term. A particular example of this is Canadian style canoeing, where a repetitive forced movement is performed completely on one side. In cycling there is a constant stretch on the ligamentous structures and joint capsules of the back causing both upper and lower back strain conditions. Running on hard surfaces causes a repetitive jerking which mostly affects the lower back. In jumping there is a heavier jerking effect with landing, and at the same time the lower back is stretched, making it even more vulnerable. In motor racing there is often a poor sitting position and constant vibration has harmful effects especially on the discs. With these activities the sportsman should pay particular attention to posture and should take measures to prevent excessive muscle imbalance and tension.

Deep muscles of the spine

The deepest muscle layers of the back are the transverso spinal (semispinal, multifidus and rotator muscles), interspinal and intertransverse muscles. They attach to the spinous and transverse processes of the vertebrae, running from one vertebrae to the next, or running across several. The deep muscles bend the spine backward, sideways and rotate it. They coordinate motion between the vertebrae. These structures make the back muscles extremely strong.

Many back and neck disorders and traumas affect facet (synovial) joints, ligaments, discs and these deep muscles. They often cause local muscle tension and tenderness when palpated. In sportsmen this local primary dysfunction is often the result of accumulated tension due to intensive training and inadequate recovery of the back from it. This builds up often unnoticed or with minor symptoms, allowing training to continue normally. If there is not impact trauma or structural fault the real cause is often with bad postural habits or poor sports technique. Wrong technique may only be apparent with efforts near the maximal capacity. There is often restricted movement locally in some areas of the back. Characteristically movement is restricted and painful only in some directions and may be perfectly normal in others. These conditions are most effectively treated by mobilisation and manipulation directed specifically to the affected area of the back with additional exercises specifically planned for the individual. Traction can sometimes be helpful, if the equipment is modern and if it can be applied in different directions. However, it may make the condition even worse if just given as a matter of routine treatment for back pain and always done in the same direction without taking into account individual variations on injuries. Massage does not directly affect the deep back muscles due to overlying thick muscle layers. With deep stroking and pressure techniques one can however often induce relaxation in them by releasing tension in the erector muscles.

Erector muscles of the spine

These muscles (iliocostal, longissimus and spinal muscles) originate from the iliac crest, spinous processes, transverse processes and angles of the ribs. They insert into the angles of the ribs, transverse and spinous processes. They extend and laterally flex the spine. During lifting they stabilise the spine with the deep back muscles, if the spine is not allowed to bend forwards too much.

Injuries in the deep structures cause stiffening in superficial back muscles. With long-standing cases, deep traumas may have healed but painful spasm in the superficial muscles can still remain. This

can be effectively treated with massage. When massage achieves relaxation in the superficial muscles, the deep layers will also gradually become more relaxed. In acute strains or sprains of deep structures of the back, massage can be performed two to three days after acute treatment (cold pack and rest). If massage is applied too early it merely causes irritation and increases muscle tension and pain. As a postacute treatment it may be sufficient to

Deep longitudinal stroking using the pads of both thumbs, supporting each other, on the same side of the spine treating the erector spinae muscle. Strokes start over the ligaments on the sacral bone or, if this area is extremely tender, one can start a little higher up. Treatment should be applied slowly in short sections to avoid excessive pain, especially in cases of lower back pain

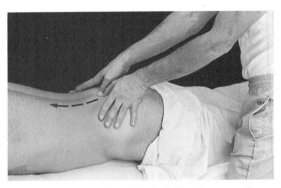

Deep transverse stroking using both thumbs supporting each other and working laterally across the erector spinae muscle. Treatment is started from the lower back or a less tender area higher up

Superficial stroking using the palms of the hands in an upwards direction along the erector spinae muscles

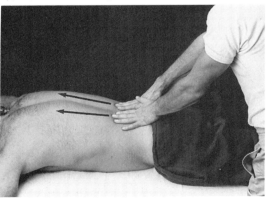

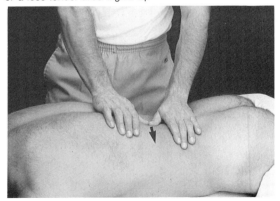

68

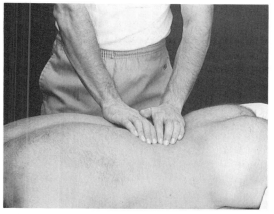

Using the fingers to apply deep pressure to the lateral border of the erector spinae muscle group, to induce relaxation when the muscles are too tense to effectively apply deep stroking. This picture also shows acupressure therapy for the urinary bladder channel, which should be treated always with back pain conditions

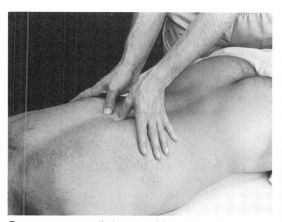

Deep pressure applied on the sides of the spinous processes, then applying a stroke up to the intervertebral spaces. This stretches the superficial fascia and skin and is used to induce reflectory relaxation. It is regularly used in connective tissue therapy

abolish pain and induce relaxation. If there is not a disc prolapse the sportsman should, with proper treatment, have regained normal active movement within a week and can return to normal training gradually within the following two weeks. Maximal efforts should be possible about a month after the onset of the injury. Failure

to obtain improvement when treating back problems may be because there is still deep irritative damage (fracture, disc prolapse) or structures like scar tissue may have formed, causing pain and limited movement. This may not be obvious if movement is not tested segmentally as other parts of the back may well compensate for a local restriction. In these cases segmental mobilisation should be performed by a person who has specialised in this kind of treatment. Another common reason is that the sportsman may return to training too soon or begin it too intensively, causing further trauma.

Quadratus lumborum muscle

This muscle originates from the transverse processes of L1-4 and the 12th rib, it attaches to the iliac crest and iliolumbar ligament. It bends the back sideways and draws the ribcage downwards. It is an accessory expiratory muscle being active with the abdominal muscles.

It is strained in similar sports to those which affect other back muscles, and posture is also an important factor in causing painful conditions. Pain is felt mainly locally and may simulate pain coming from the kidneys. As a superficial muscle it is easy to treat by deep stroking, but requires knowledge of special treatment position. This is because in the prone lying position it becomes too relaxed and passes easily under the treating hands.

The following are commonly used 'diagnoses' in back disorders:

Lumbago

This is a term commonly given to lower back pain without consideration of which particular structures are affected. In facet joint dysfunction and ligament sprains recovery will be quickly obtained through

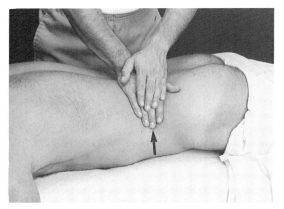

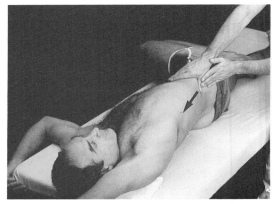

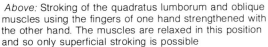

Above: Stroking of the quadratus lumborum and oblique muscles using the fingers of one hand strengthened with the other hand. The muscles are relaxed in this position and so only superficial stroking is possible

Above right: The sportsman is in the supine position, but with the pelvis rotated through 90 degrees and the upper hip flexed. The knee is also flexed and the foot rests on the back of the knee of the other leg, providing stability. The arm on the same side is brought up beside the head. In this position the quadratus lumborum and oblique muscles are stretched and easy to reach. Problem areas can be identified as they do not easily slide away under the hands. Deep stroking is applied with the thumb and is reinforced with the other hand on the lateral border of the quadratus lumborum muscle

Right: Deep stroking along the intercostal muscles using the fingers of one hand reinforced with the overlying hand

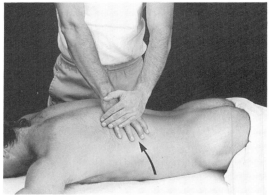

manipulative treatment. Without it recovery is delayed and sometimes chronic painful conditions may develop as there will be degeneration in the structures from being immobilised for a long time. This would never be allowed with joints, for example, in arms and legs, but unfortunately it often happens with joints of the back.

Sciatica

This refers to low back pain, which radiates down the leg. It is a term often used in conjunction with 'slipped disc', and indeed a prolapsed disc can cause such symptoms by pinching the nerve root. However, it is far more often caused by facet joint dysfunction, ligament tears and segmental muscle tension in areas surrounding the trauma. This explains why one can often get good results with massage in back disorders like 'sciatica'. A prolapsed disc is not a contraindication for massage. On the contrary, the therapist is often able to give great relief by relaxing secondary muscle tension.

THE SHOULDERS (see also pp. 78–9)

Many painful conditions can develop in the shoulders, upper back and neck, which can lead to diffused aching or weakness in the arms. This is often vertebrogenic in origin, and sometimes in chronic shoulder conditions it may be caused by a disturbance in the autonomic nervous system.

This can give rise to increased muscle tension, radiated pain to the arm, diffused tenderness, decline in temperature and even atrophy. If effective, early treatment is not given, recovery can take a long time.

Greater and lesser rhomboid muscles

These muscles run from C6-7 (lesser) and T1-4 (greater) spinous processes to the medial side of the shoulder blade. Their action is to draw back and to rotate the shoulder blade.

The rhomboid muscles may become strained in sports like rowing, canoeing and skiing. Pain is usually felt locally, but it may radiate to the front of the chest, and a sharp piercing sensation may be experienced through the area. Aching in these muscles is common with thoracic vertebral joint dysfunction due to postural strain. In such conditions mobilisation and manipulation treatment should be considered. Excessive tension can develop in the rhomboids due to poor posture, and is more common in sportsmen who are also affected by occupational stress, such as working behind a desk. Massage releases tension in them and also often induces relaxation in deeper muscles of the vertebral column.

With the arm rotated inwards and resting on the back causing the vertebral border of the scapula to be raised upwards. This is to expose the attachments of the muscle. Deep longitudinal stroking can be applied with the thumb strengthened by the other hand along the course of the rhomboid muscles from the attachment on the shoulder blade to the spine

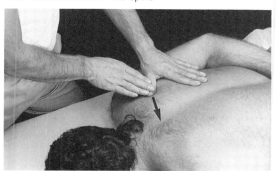

Deltoid muscle

The deltoid muscle arises in the clavicle, the acromion process and spine of the scapula. It extends to the deltoid tuberosity of the humerus. Its action is to lift the upper arm in all possible directions.

The deltoid may become overstrained in any sport involving strenuous arm movement above the level of the shoulder, particularly racket sports and weight lifting, and usually affects the anterior part.

Deep stroking of the deltoid muscle using the pads of both thumbs together. The direction of the strokes is upwards. The therapist should, however, stop before the acromion to avoid crushing the muscles on the bone. Instead one should make short strokes downwards, starting from the insertion on the acromion process of the scapula

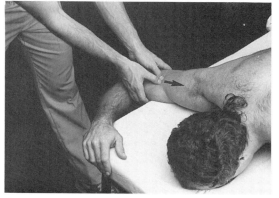

With the elbow flexed and resting on the therapist's thigh, both hands can be used to apply kneading to the belly of the deltoid muscle

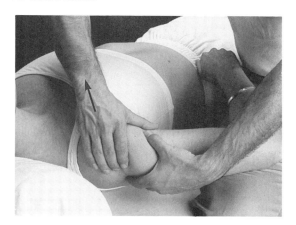

Occasionally the middle part of the muscle is strained and pain has a less definite location. Trauma normally affects the muscle near the attachment with the humerus on the lateral side in the middle of the upper arm. The deltoid is an easy muscle to treat with massage and responds well to deep stroking and friction.

Supraspinatus muscle

This muscle has its origin in the supraspinous fossa of the scapula and inserts into the greater tuberosity of the humerus. Its action is to abduct the arm.

Tendinitis towards the attachment of this muscle is a common cause of severe shoulder pain. It is often found in sports which involve a sudden high strain on the shoulder, like javelin and shot put or weight lifting. It can also occur in sports which require repetitive movement with the arm raised above the shoulder like in swimming (particularly backstroke and crawl) and racket sports. Typically pain appears in a certain range of abduction (sixty to 120 degrees) as the traumatised supraspinatus tendon becomes trapped

With the arm maximally adducted resting comfortably across the back the supraspinatus muscle is relaxed and in a good position for massage. The thumb strengthened by the other hand is used to apply deep longitudinal stroking to it

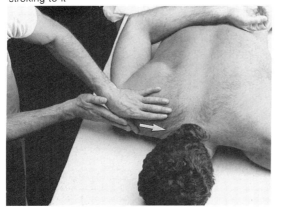

against the acromion and corococromial ligaments by the head of the humerus. Pain may radiate down the arm and sometimes even imitate 'tennis elbow'. The subdeltoid bursa often becomes inflamed, and the whole shoulder may sometimes be swollen with supraspinatus tendinitis. As other muscles around the shoulder become tense in this condition, diagnosis is not always clear. In acute cases, providing tendon rupture has been ruled out, the best thing is to apply massage one or two times to the whole shoulder area, after applying cold packs. This should relax the surrounding muscles and enable better diagnosis. Deep friction to the attachment has often proved to be more irritative than beneficial. The tendon cannot be reached with massage as it runs beneath the acromion. Tension pain in the supraspinatus muscle and trigger points may simulate the symptoms of supraspinatus tendinitis, but in these cases it may be completely treated with just a few massage treatments.

Infraspinatus and teres minor muscles

These muscles arise in the infraspinous fossa of the scapula and insert into the greater tuberosity of the humerus, and their action is to rotate the arm outwards.

Painful conditions appear in throwing sports, racket sports, body building and other weight training. The muscles are liable to strain when the arm is moved quickly up and backwards. Pain from the teres minor is felt more locally near its attachment to the humerus, and from the infraspinatus it is often felt in the belly of the muscle. It may radiate down the lateral side of the arm, even to the fingers. Pain around the shoulder is diffused and often difficult to localise, but can be felt more often in the front of the shoulder joint. Pain from these muscles makes it difficult to rotate the arm inwards and to reach up

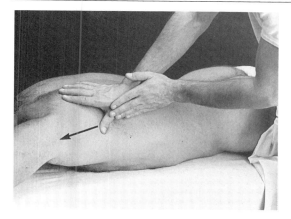

With the arm brought up on the side of the head the infraspinatus, teres major, teres minor and distal part of the latissimus dorsi muscles are stretched. Deep stroking is applied with the thumb reinforced with the other hand. This position allows the therapist to direct treatment more specifically to these different muscles. While treating the infraspinatus muscle one should keep in mind the course of the muscle and not push it against the spine of the scapula

When the arm is in an upward position these muscles pull the arm downwards and so are vulnerable to injury in sports like mountain climbing, throwing sports and pole vault. The latissimus dorsi is a much bigger and stronger muscle working a longer lever than teres major and goes round it before attaching jointly to the humerus. The teres minor is a much smaller muscle having a shorter range and

The shoulder is stretched upwards by pulling the arm. Deep transverse stroking is applied with the thumb of the other hand to stretch the tendons of the latissimus dorsi and teres major muscles, which become more accessible in this position

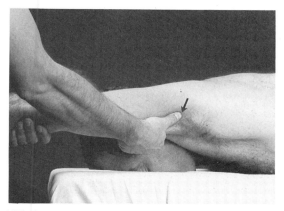

With the arm brought up on the side of the head the palmar surface of the thumb can be used to apply stroking and squeezing to the upper part of the latissimus dorsi muscle. It also provides a good position for treating the subscapularis muscle under the scapula

across the back to touch the other shoulder blade which causes acute pain as the traumatised muscle becomes stretched. This may therefore simulate 'frozen shoulder' syndrome, where adhesive capsulitis of the shoulder joint can cause a limitation of movement. The difference in the two is important as massage gives good quick results with musculotendinous trauma, but with capsulitis it is only beneficial for relieving secondary muscle tension and more emphasis has to be put on mobilisation.

Latissimus dorsi and teres major muscles

The latissimus dorsi has its origin in the spinous processes of Th7-12 and through the lumbodorsal fascia to the lumbar vertebrae and iliac crest. The teres major arises in the inferior angle of the scapula. They both attach to the lesser tubercle of the humerus. Their action is to draw the arm backwards, rotate it inwards and assist in adduction.

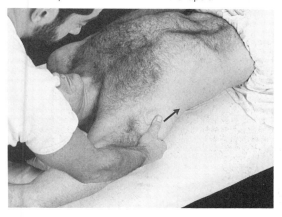

is therefore more prone to strains, which are usually located near the attachment with the upper arm. This area is often neglected in treatment, which usually concentrates on the belly of the muscle. There is secondary tension and radiated pain felt in the muscle belly, but treatment there gives only temporary and partial improvement. All parts of these muscles can be easily reached by massage with deep stroking to the muscle, and friction near the attachment should be applied in traumas.

Subscapularis muscle

This muscle runs from the medial inner surface of the scapula to the lesser tuberosity on the front side of the humerus. It is the strongest inward rotator of the arm.

The subscapularis muscle is subject to strain in throwing sports, particularly discus and javelin, as well as baseball and racket sports. Overuse strain can occur from repetitive arm movements, but is often caused due to a technical fault causing excessive outward rotation of the humerus, which has to be counteracted by the subscapularis. Excessive tension can

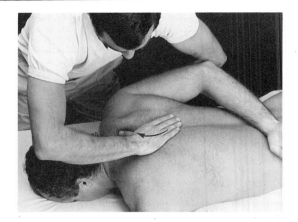

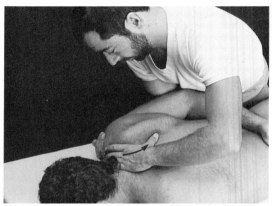

Top: With the arm inwardly rotated and resting across the back, the therapist grasps the shoulder and lifts it upwards with his forearm. The thumb on the other hand can apply deep stroking to the upper part of the subscapularis muscle and insertion of the levator scapulae muscle. It also stretches the rhomboid muscle at the same time

Middle: The therapist grasps the front side of the shoulder using his forearm to lift the arm and shoulder. The thumb is used to apply deep stroking to the lower part of subscapularis muscle and stretches the rhomboid muscle

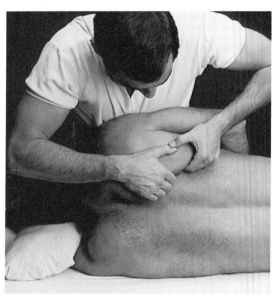

Bottom: In a side lying position, with knees and hips bent to maintain the position. The arm is hanging relaxed across the front of the body and the shoulder and upper arm are supported against the therapist. The therapist puts his fingers in the vertebral border of the scapulae and leans forwards in order to get the scapula to move over the fingers. One should have a firm grasp deeply under the scapula and then lift it outwards to stretch the subscapularis and rhomboideus muscles

often develop, which may lead to severe shoulder trauma. The subscapularis is the first muscle to tense up in cases of adhesive capsulitis of the shoulder joint (frozen shoulder), and outward rotation of the arm can become severely restricted. Other muscles will stiffen up, but only later on in the condition. Pain is referred to the back of the shoulder blade, so if treatment is given according to the symptoms it will not be very effective. The belly of the muscle is reached by lifting the scapula, but this may require great effort with sportsmen of stocky build. The most effective part of treatment is deep friction massage applied to the attachment near the arm. Early treatment of this condition is important as it is likely otherwise to become chronic and take a long time to rehabilitate.

THE NECK (see illustrations on pp. 78–9)

The muscles of the neck are prone to injury in many sports. The muscles tense up unilaterally in sports which predominantly use one arm, particularly throwing events like shot put, (table) tennis and racket sports. If muscle development is controlled and excessive strain is avoided during training this does not necessarily cause any problems. In endurance sports, like running and walking, the neck muscles tend to remain in isometric contraction for long periods as the sportsman tries to achieve maximal effort. This is because the shoulders are kept up in order to make breathing more easy as the ribcage is allowed to widen more freely on inhalation. It is, however, better to try to relax them consciously as this will allow expiration to happen fully, which is just as important. In cycling the neck is held in extension for long periods, and in particular the sub-occipital muscles have a tendency to remain in tight contraction. In all outdoor sports the neck muscles are often exposed to wind, cold and damp, which causes tension in the muscles. If the tension is not released from time to time it can become a chronic condition.

Trapezius muscle

This muscle originates at the occipital bone and all the cervical and thoracic spinous processes and inserts into the clavicle and scapula spine. It is the most superficial of all the muscles of the upper back and neck. Its action is to elevate, lower, rotate and brace the scapula. The trapezius also rotates the head and bends it backwards.

Stiffness and tension result in pain felt in the shoulders, between the shoulder blades and in the neck. Chronic tension can build up at the occipital attachment and is often related to poor posture. Thoracic kyphosis can cause the muscle in this area to contract in a similar way to that in cycling described above. Also bad postural habits like shrinking down while relaxing, especially when sitting, causes stretching in the back muscles and the neck muscles become tense as they have to bend backwards to maintain an upright head position. Pain may not always be felt locally, but may cause frontal and tem-

Deep transverse stroking applied to the belly of the trapezius muscle, using the fingers of one hand strengthened by the other hand

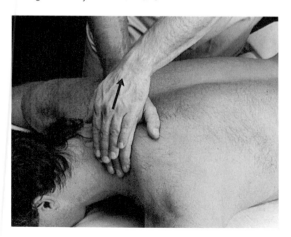

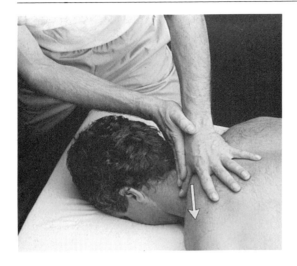

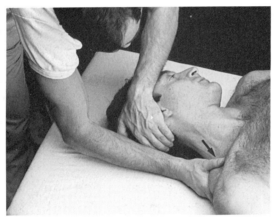

Top: Deep longitudinal stroking performed on the trapezius muscle, using the thumb of one hand strengthened by the other hand

Above: Using one hand to hold the head in a sidebent position away from the side being treated and to apply stretch to the trapezius muscle, deep longitudinal stroking is applied to the front part of it

poral headaches. Over eighty per cent of headaches originate from neck and masticatory muscles, and often tension in them is combined. From the lateral part of the trapezius muscle pain may radiate to the radial side of the forearm. Transverse stroking is applied to the muscle and deep pressure should be applied along the occipital attachment to release tension.

Levator scapulae, splenius muscle of the head and neck

These all locate under the trapezius muscle. The levator scapulae originates from the upper four cervical vertebrae, which have the greatest range of movement in the neck. It inserts into the upper medial part of the scapulae, and elevates and rotates it. The splenius muscles originate from the spinous processes C4–Th5 and insert into the mastoid process and behind it. They bend the head backwards and rotate it.

The levator scapulae is the main muscle involved with neck pain, due to strenuous training, which is felt diffusely in the neck and shoulder. The levator is under tension all the time the arms are working. Problems in the splenius muscles cause similar symptoms to those with the trapezius muscle with neck pain and headaches. These muscles can still be easily reached with massage. Deep pressure applied near the levators attachment to the scapulae effectively relieves tension in the neck muscles.

Deep pressure is applied with the thumb supported by the other hand at the attachment of the levator scapula muscle to the scapula to induce effective relaxation

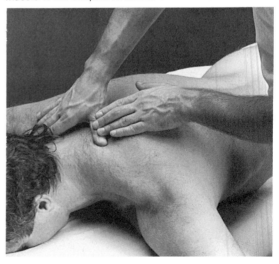

76

In acute injuries pain is mostly felt locally in the affected part of the neck and occipital area. From the upper cervicals pain is often referred to the head, causing temporal and frontal headache. A middle cervical strain may cause referred pain to the shoulders, and lower strains can go to the arms. Entrapment of the greater occipital nerve due to tension in the semispinalis capitis muscle may cause tingling and numbness in the occipital region. Local trauma in the neck may cause problems in the lower spine as this is a balanced structure in which the function of the parts are dependent on each other. Even though these are deep muscles the superficial muscle layer is not as thick as in the back, and deep transverse stroking is an effective way to release muscle tension.

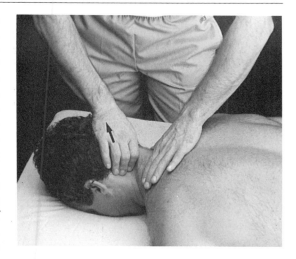

The deep posterior neck muscles

These muscles (semispinalis, capitis and cervicis, longissimus, multifidi, rotatores and suboccipital muscles) form the closest layer to the facet joints. Their function is to direct the movement between the vertebrae, rotate the neck and bend it backwards. They are the first muscles to tense up with local trauma and postural problems in the joints or adjacent structures.

The deep muscles are relatively small in relation to the load on top of the neck and they are liable to strain if subjected to sudden forced movement (whiplash injury).

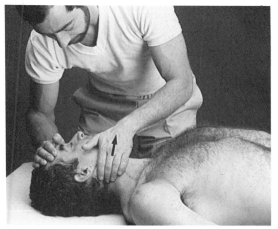

Top right: Deep transverse stroking to the neck muscles, applied with the fingers and thumbs of both hands alternately. One should apply strokes slowly when there is a painful condition or excessive tension, to avoid irritation

Middle right: Using one hand to steady the head in a slightly rotated position away from the side being treated, the fingers of the other hand can be used to apply transverse stroking to the neck muscles

Bottom right: Using the tips of the fingers, deep pressure is applied on the attachments of the deep cervical muscles under the occiput

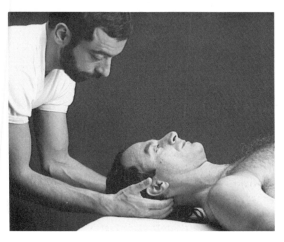

Superficial muscles　　　　　　　　**Bones**

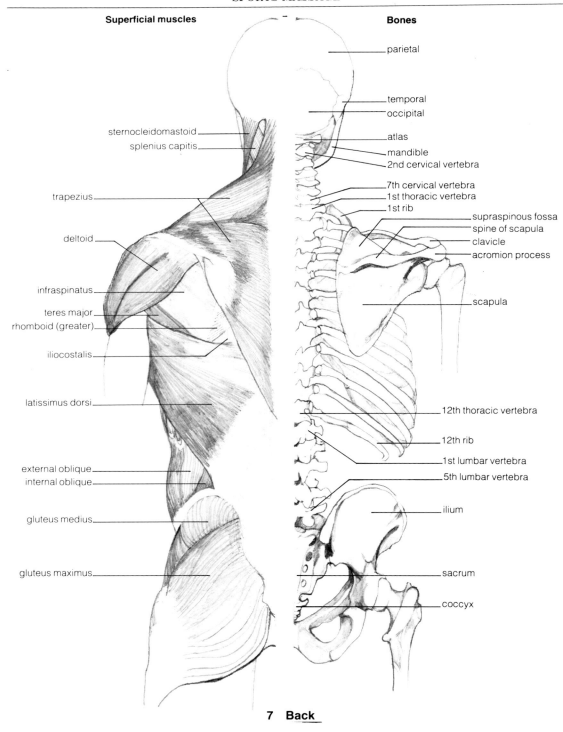

parietal

temporal
occipital

sternocleidomastoid
splenius capitis

atlas
mandible
2nd cervical vertebra

trapezius

7th cervical vertebra
1st thoracic vertebra
1st rib
supraspinous fossa
spine of scapula
clavicle
acromion process

deltoid

infraspinatus

scapula

teres major
rhomboid (greater)

iliocostalis

latissimus dorsi

12th thoracic vertebra

12th rib
1st lumbar vertebra
5th lumbar vertebra

external oblique
internal oblique

ilium

gluteus medius

gluteus maximus

sacrum

coccyx

7　Back

Deep muscles

Bones

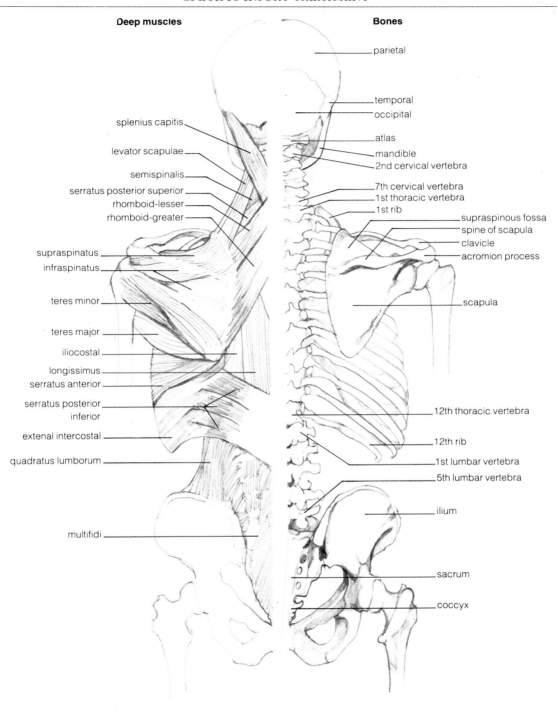

splenius capitis

levator scapulae

semispinalis

serratus posterior superior

rhomboid-lesser

rhomboid-greater

supraspinatus

infraspinatus

teres minor

teres major

iliocostal

longissimus

serratus anterior

serratus posterior
inferior

extenal intercostal

quadratus lumborum

multifidi

parietal

temporal

occipital

atlas

mandible

2nd cervical vertebra

7th cervical vertebra

1st thoracic vertebra

1st rib

supraspinous fossa

spine of scapula

clavicle

acromion process

scapula

12th thoracic vertebra

12th rib

1st lumbar vertebra

5th lumbar vertebra

ilium

sacrum

coccyx

8 Back

Acute neck strains are common in contact sports like rugby and American football. In motor sports the neck may be strained as a result of a collision with another vehicle. In cycling, due to falling off at speed, the neck is vulnerable, even though the head is protected with a helmet.

Scalenus muscles (anterior, medius and posterior)

The main scalenus muscles are the anterior, which runs from transverse processes C3-6, and medius C2-7, and they attach to the first rib. The medial and posterior muscles run similarly. Their action is to bend the head laterally and rotate it. They also lift the first rib, being active therefore in inspiration.

The scalenus muscles tense up especially in weight lifting and are under considerable strain in powerlifting. Carrying bags causes isometric contraction to them. Excessive tension can develop easily due to bad posture or physical stress in combina-

Using one hand to hold the head in a rotated position away from the side being treated, to stretch the scalenus muscles. This position will allow deep stroking techniques to be applied without causing pressure to underlying sensitive structures, especially the cervical artery. The thumb is used to apply longitudinal stroking to the scalenus muscles

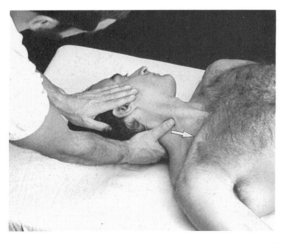

tion with tension in other neck muscles and is therefore seen in many different sports. Pain from these muscles is usually felt in the back of the neck and remains unnoticed in the front. Symptoms may also be felt in the shoulders and arms. Muscle tension can cause compression on the subclavian artery and entrapment of the brachial plexus as they pass between the scalenus anterior and medius muscles. Referred pain from the muscles may be felt in the radial side of the hand. Entrapment of the brachial plexus may cause pain in the ulnar side of the hand, with sensation of pins and needles or even sensory loss and weakness in the arm (thoracic outlet syndrome).

Massage treatment for neck pains often show poor results because the treatment is performed only on the muscles at the back side of the neck. The muscles in the front are of equal importance and should not be neglected. When treating these muscles care must be taken to avoid putting pressure on sensitive structures. The cervical artery and thyroid gland should not be compressed. This can be done without missing out on effective massage by turning the head away from the side being worked on. This stretches the scalenus muscles and makes it possible to apply deep stroking techniques without applying pressure on the structures beneath.

Sternocleidomastoid muscle

This muscle has its origin in the sternum and clavicle and travels up to insert into the mastoid process of the temporal bone. It flexes the neck backwards and rotates the head to the opposite side.

The muscle is subject to strain in all walks of life and is not related to any specific sport. Tension often goes together with that in the scalenus muscles. Similarly, pain is seldom felt locally and may be referred to the temporal and frontal areas.

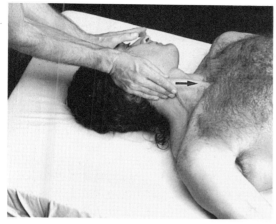

Using one hand to fix the head in a rotated position away from the side being treated, the thumb and fingers of the other hand are used to grasp the sides of the sternocleidomastoid muscle, and to apply longitudinal stroking and stretching. One should use only short gentle strokes as it is often tender particularly with neck troubles

Stiffness is felt locally when the head is moved in the opposite direction, but to catch the source of pain one has to search for trigger points. Treatment should always be carried out on it together with the scalenus muscles.

THE ARMS (see illustrations on pp. 86-9)

Biceps muscle

The biceps brachii muscle has two parts. The long one has its origin at the scapula above the axillary joint, and its tendon passes through the joint capsule. The short head attaches to the coracoid process of the scapula. They inset into the radius and ulna via a strong two headed tendon. The biceps assists in shoulder joint flexion, but its main action is to flex the elbow joint. When the elbow is bent, it has a stronger effect on rotating the lower arm outwards than the supinator muscle. This movement can be used as a resisted test to check for inflammation in the tendon of the long head.

The biceps muscle commonly suffers overstrain in sports involving powerful flexion of the arm, like in mountain climbing, wrestling and weight lifting. Strains may occur at the end of rapid throwing movements, for example striking the ball in racket sports and blocking in volleyball. The tendon of the long head is more commonly injured than that of the short head. From tenderness found by

Holding the lower arm in an elevated position to ensure the biceps muscle is fully relaxed. The thumb and fingers of the other hand are used to apply longitudinal stroking

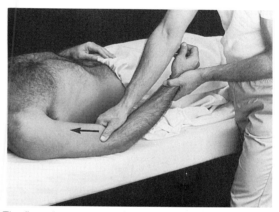

The fingertips are used to apply deep friction to the tendon of the long head of the biceps muscle running in a groove between two tubercles of the humerus. Friction may also be applied: to the medial side to treat the insertion of the internal rotator muscles, or the lateral side to treat the insertion of the outward rotator muscles of the shoulder joint

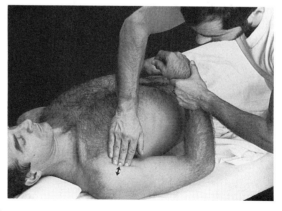

palpation along its course between the tubercles at the proximal end of the humerus it is difficult to diagnose which structure is affected. The internal and external rotators of the shoulder attach to the lesser and greater tubercles, respectively. There are many attachments of muscles close to one another, which makes it difficult to identify the correct source of the problem. Resisted muscle tests should be used to find the cause of the pain. Pain from the muscle belly may be referred to the shoulder joint, and is the most common disorder for the biceps. Good results can be obtained with massage of the muscle and deep friction to the tendons.

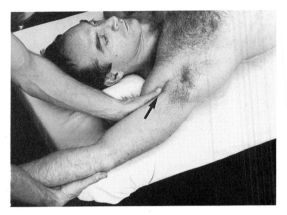

The arm is brought up beside the head to induce a stretch to the coracobrachialis muscle and to better expose the proximal part of it. Deep friction can be applied using the thumb

Coracobrachialis muscle

This muscle arises from the coracoid process of the scapula and attaches along the shaft of the humerus, and it draws the arm forwards and medially.

Strains mainly occur in racket sports, and pain is usually felt towards the shoulder. The muscle is overlapped by the pectoralis major and deltoid muscles, making it easy to mistakenly treat the wrong area. Similar symptoms can develop if there is a problem affecting the short head

Holding the arm in a slightly abducted and outwardly rotated position, deep longitudinal stroking is applied with the thumb to the coracobrachialis muscle

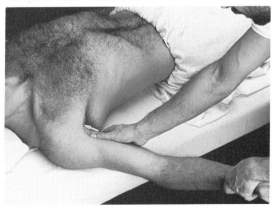

of the biceps which attaches to the coracoid process just medial to the coracobrachialis. Massage treatment is very effective, but care must be taken to apply deep friction exactly on the site of any trauma if it is to be successful.

Triceps muscle

This muscle has three parts: the long head attaching to the scapula and the medial and lateral heads to the humerus. It inserts by a strong tendon into the olecranon of the ulna. Fibres from the triceps muscle attach to the capsule of the elbow joint (articular muscle of the elbow). It is the strongest muscle of the arm, it extends the elbow, stretches the joint capsule and helps extend the shoulder.

The triceps muscle is under strain in sports like weight lifting, boxing, shot put, javelin and other throwing sports. Overuse strain can cause radiated pain upwards to the shoulder and downwards to the hand on the ulnar side. Pain is often felt inside of the elbow joint because the triceps has a direct connection with it. The symptoms may not appear during normal activity but

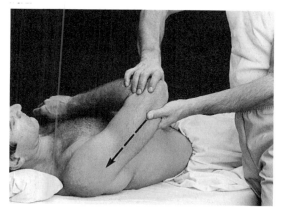

The arm is held in an elevated position with the elbow flexed and supported with one hand. The fingers and thumb of the other hand are used to apply deep stroking on the triceps muscle. Special attention should be given to the part near the olecranon

is usually localised, but may also be referred into the hand, especially on the radial side. With deep friction the tight muscle bands can be released and the symptoms may disappear completely.

Brachioradialis muscle

This muscle has its origin above the lateral epicondyle of the humerus and attaches to the styloid process of the radius. It is the only muscle in the forearm which acts on a single joint, the elbow. Due to its location, a painful condition may imitate tennis elbow but will respond more easily to treatment. Radiated pain may be felt in the radial side of the wrist.

only when effort is applied. This referred pain can be relieved by deep friction massage applied on the local trauma.

Excessive muscle tension or trauma can cause compression to the radial nerve, causing pain, numbness and pins and needles sensations on the radial side of the hand. The whole arm may ache in combination with referred pain from the muscle and radial nerve irritation. This can be treated by massage and stretching.

Brachialis muscle

This muscle has its origin along the shaft of the humerus and attaches to the coracoid process and tuberosity of the ulna. Its function is in flexion of the elbow joint.

If the brachialis muscle is well developed and stiff due to training, and if one sleeps with the arm forcefully flexed underneath the body, entrapment of the radial nerve can sometimes result. Pain, numbness and pins and needles may be felt in the hand, particularly at the root of the thumb. There may also be weakness in the extensor muscles in the forearm. Pain caused by excessive tension in the brachialis muscle

With the forearm held in an elevated position so the elbow is slightly flexed and the brachialis muscle is relaxed. The fingers apply deep transverse stroking to the brachialis muscle

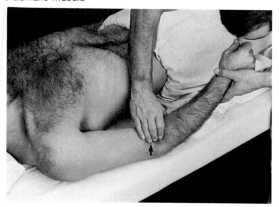

The extensor muscles of the wrist and fingers

The long and short radial extensor muscle of the wrist, common extensor muscle of fingers and extensor muscle of little finger originate from the lateral epicondyle of the humerus and insert into the bones of the wrist and fingers.

Overstrain is the main problem affecting the forearm muscles, and they are most at risk in sports which involve repetitive arm movements while the hand is kept in isometric contraction, usually when holding a piece of equipment. Therefore the high risk sports with this problem include tennis, squash and other racket sports, golf, canoeing and rowing. The continual contraction of the hand causes a restriction in circulation and so recovery often remains incomplete if no therapy is applied. It therefore has a great tendency to develop gradually into a chronic problem, and, to prevent this, treatment should be given at the first sign of pain or stiffness. Rest alone is seldom an effective treatment as it may only give temporary symptom relief.

Pain from these muscles is mainly referred to the wrist and fingers, tending to be more on the side in which they insert. Excessive tension in the extensor carpi radialis brevis and its fascia may exert pressure on the radial nerve, causing the same effects as described with the brachialis muscle, and should be treated similarly.

The condition called 'tennis elbow' (lateral epicondylitis) is the most common problem affecting the forearm. It is found not just in tennis players but in many other sportsmen as indicated above, and also affects many people not involved in sport, for example in occupations such as carpentry and typing, and in leisure activities like gardening and knitting. Pain is felt at the lateral side of the elbow joint and can be very intense, resulting in limited function of the wrist and hand. Pain can radiate up into the shoulder and down to the whole arm and hand because several muscles can be involved. In chronic conditions muscle tension may even be found in the flexor side of the forearm. The problem arises in the lateral epicondyle of the elbow, where the extensor muscles of the wrist and fingers and supinator muscle attach. Excessive tension or trauma can

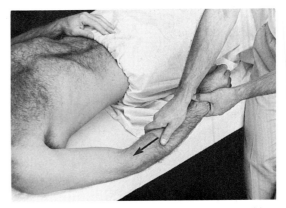

Holding the forearm in an elevated and inward rotated position from the wrist, the fingers and thumb apply longitudinal stroking from the wrist to the elbow along the extensor muscles of the forearm

cause strain and inflammation on the attachment of the common extensor tendon. Problems in one or several extensor muscles can be the cause of tennis elbow so the whole area should be massaged thoroughly. Early treatment is very important: massage and cold packs should be applied, and also ultrasound has been shown to be effective. The main aim in massage is to release tension in the whole extensor muscle area, release adhesions and improve the circulation.

Therapists are at risk of getting tennis elbow themselves through doing massage and should perform regular self massage to prevent tension building up in the forearm. People in sports which have a high incidence of tennis elbow, or who have a history of this condition, should also be taught how to give local effective self massage treatment.

The abductor pollicus longus, extensor pollicus longus and brevis muscles

These originate from the mid forearm, dorsal surface of the ulna, radius and interosseus membrane running to the thumb. They function according to their names.

The commonest problem with these muscles is a tendency to develop tenosynovitis. This is due to overstrain from repetitive movements and continuous isometric contraction, and is common in sports like canoeing and racket sports. It may also occur in therapists who do a lot of massage and continually forget to give self treatment. Pain is felt in the radial side of the wrist where there also may be swelling. In acute cases crepitation may be felt on palpation. Pain may radiate to the thumb and up the forearm. Massage should be applied with deep friction across the course of the tendon to improve circulation, prevent adhesions and to relieve pain. Similar conditions can occur on the flexor side, but are far less common. Treatment should be applied in the same way.

Supinator muscle

This muscle is located in the deep layer of the proximal part of the forearm, and arises at the lateral epicondyle of the humerus and dorsal surface of the ulna. It inserts along the frontal and lateral surface of the radius. The supinator muscle attaches also to the lateral collateral and annular ligaments of the elbow, stretching them. Its action is to supinate the forearm, which can be used for muscle testing to provoke pain.

Aching due to strain on the muscle is felt at the lateral epicondyle and is a common cause of lateral epicondylitis (tennis elbow). Other muscles are usually also involved and this condition is described above. Pain

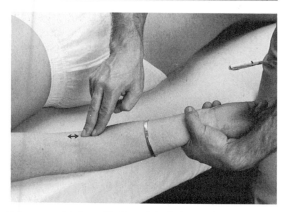

Deep cross friction with tips of the index and middle fingers are applied on the supinator muscle

from the supinator muscle may be felt at the base of the thumb on the back side of the hand. Stiffness in the supinator muscle can cause compression on the radial nerve, giving rise to entrapment syndrome below the lateral epicondyle. It may appear in combination with tennis elbow, complicating diagnosis and treatment. When the arm is supinated weakness is typically found in the wrist and finger extension. Symptoms are the same as those described with the triceps muscle which can also cause entrapment. To obtain good results with treatment, massage must be deep enough to reach the target through the superficial layer. Manipulation and deep stroking will relieve the muscle tension.

Round pronator muscle, wrist and finger flexor muscles

Round pronator muscle, radial and ulnar flexor muscles of the wrist and superficial flexor muscle of fingers all originate in the medial epicondyle of the humerus. The pronator muscle inserts to the middle of the external surface of radius. The flexor muscles attach to the bones of the wrist and fingers. They function according to their names.

Superficial muscles

Bones

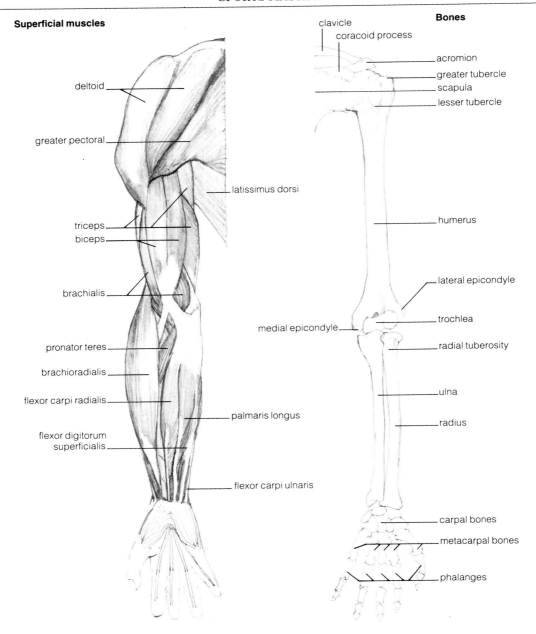

clavicle

coracoid process

acromion

greater tubercle

scapula

lesser tubercle

deltoid

greater pectoral

latissimus dorsi

humerus

triceps

biceps

brachialis

lateral epicondyle

medial epicondyle

trochlea

radial tuberosity

pronator teres

brachioradialis

flexor carpi radialis

palmaris longus

ulna

radius

flexor digitorum
superficialis

flexor carpi ulnaris

carpal bones

metacarpal bones

phalanges

9   Arm (front)

Deep muscles

Bones

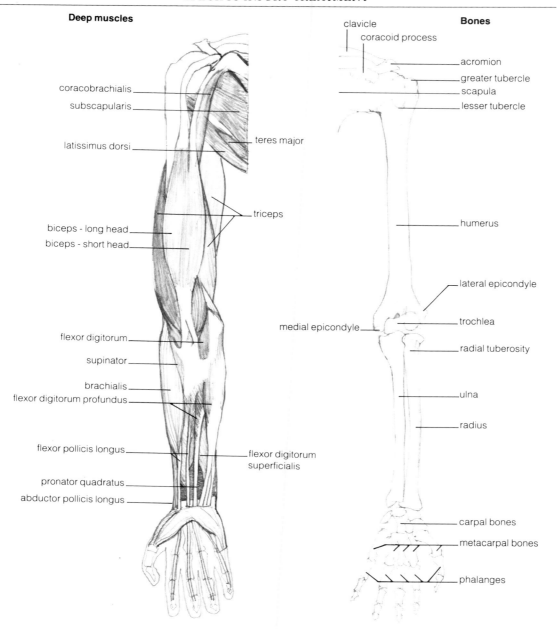

clavicle
coracoid process
acromion
greater tubercle
scapula
lesser tubercle

coracobrachialis
subscapularis

latissimus dorsi

teres major

triceps

humerus

biceps - long head
biceps - short head

lateral epicondyle

trochlea

medial epicondyle

radial tuberosity

flexor digitorum

supinator

brachialis
flexor digitorum profundus

ulna

radius

flexor pollicis longus

flexor digitorum
superficialis

pronator quadratus
abductor pollicis longus

carpal bones
metacarpal bones

phalanges

10   Arm (front)

Superficial muscles

Bones

spine of scapula
clavicle

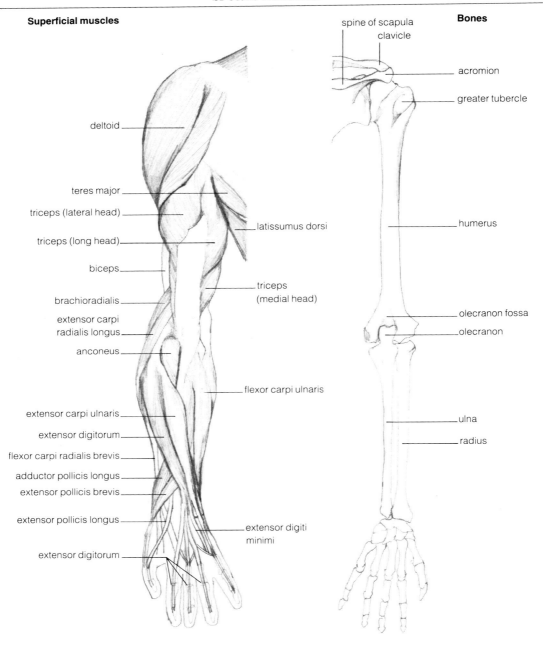

deltoid

teres major

triceps (lateral head)

triceps (long head)

biceps

brachioradialis

extensor carpi
radialis longus

anconeus

extensor carpi ulnaris

extensor digitorum

flexor carpi radialis brevis

adductor pollicis longus

extensor pollicis brevis

extensor pollicis longus

extensor digitorum

latissumus dorsi

triceps
(medial head)

flexor carpi ulnaris

extensor digiti
minimi

acromion

greater tubercle

humerus

olecranon fossa

olecranon

ulna

radius

11   Arm (back)

Deep muscles

spine of scapula
clavicle

Bones

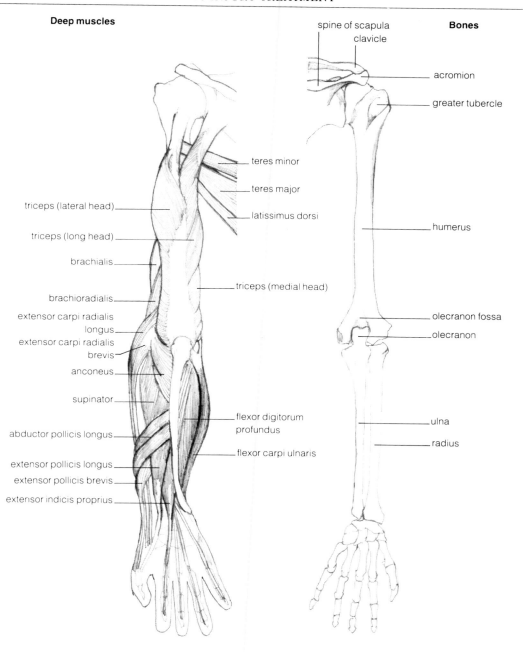

acromion

greater tubercle

teres minor

teres major

triceps (lateral head)

latissimus dorsi

triceps (long head)

humerus

brachialis

triceps (medial head)

brachioradialis

extensor carpi radialis
longus

extensor carpi radialis
brevis

olecranon fossa

olecranon

anconeus

supinator

flexor digitorum
profundus

ulna

abductor pollicis longus

radius

flexor carpi ulnaris

extensor pollicis longus

extensor pollicis brevis

extensor indicis proprius

12   Arm (back)

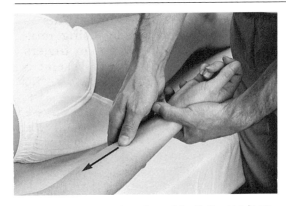

Holding the forearm up from the wrist with the arm in an outwardly rotated position, the fingers and the thumb are used to apply stroking along the forearm. This will treat the pronator teres muscle and the flexor muscles of the wrist

Epicondylitis medialis (golfers' elbow) is far less common than the corresponding condition in the lateral side. Pain is felt on the medial side of the elbow and there may be referred pain in the wrist and fingers. It may appear in sports like javelin, badminton, baseball and cricket, as well as in other throwing and racket sports. As with the extensor side, several muscles are involved. Massage should be given in the same way as described for tennis elbow. Corresponding to the extensor side, pain may radiate to the fingers from the flexor muscles and can be effectively abolished by releasing tension with deep stroking massage. The ulnar nerve runs superficially and medially down the back of the elbow and is unprotected against impact. Trauma in the cubital tunnel through which the nerve passes may develop into entrapment syndrome with numbness, pain and tingling sensations extending down the ulnar side of the forearm into the fourth and fifth fingers. It may also be caused by tension in the flexor muscles which can be relieved simply with massage. The median nerve may also be affected in the same way as it runs in front of the elbow joint and past the pronator muscles. This will cause pain down into the first to third fingers. Deep friction on the site of the entrapment and deep stroking to release tension from muscle and fascia are effective treatments.

Carpal tunnel syndrome

The median nerve may become compressed due to inflammation of the tendons passing over the wrist bones and beneath the flexor retinaculum. There is a small space there where nerves pass into the hand which may become congested by swelling of the surrounding structures. This is usually due to irritation caused by long-standing compression and is found in cycling or from repeated blows in racket and batting sports. Pain and numbness radiate down towards the first three fingers or up mainly along the lateral side of the arm. After acute treatment, and when the swelling has reduced, deep friction massage can be applied. This should be done in the same direction as the tendons and thus run across the direction of the flexor retinaculum. This is to stretch it, break adhesions and improve circulation. One has to be careful to avoid causing compression to the median nerve, which may make symptoms worse. Stretching to the wrist bones should be applied sideways (schapoid and trapezium in a radial direction and simultan-

The thumb is used to apply deep friction against the flexor retinaculum above the carpal tunnel

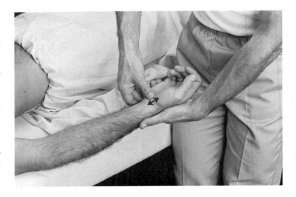

eously pisiform and hamate bones in the ulnar direction).

The hand

The adductor and opposing muscle of the thumb are of major importance in giving a firm grip. Painful conditions appear often in racket sports due to long-standing isometric contraction. Pain is felt around

With the palm of the hand resting in the fingers, the thumbs are used to apply stroking to the back of the hand

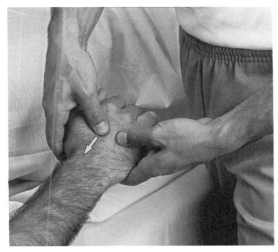

With the back of the hand resting in the fingers, the thumbs are used to apply stroking and friction to the palm area. Stretching can be performed by deep stroking with both thumbs moving sideways from each other

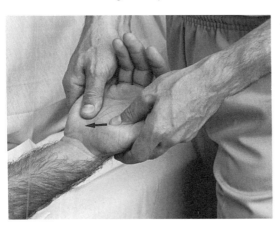

the thumb on the palmar side. This is easily treated by oneself by using rotational pressure with the thumb or fingers of the other hand. This should become a familiar practice to all sportsmen who need a strong grip.

Pain in interossei muscles of the fingers is due to long standing strain on the fingers and occurs sometimes in sports like shot put. Pain is referred along the fingers and is also easily treated.

THE CHEST (see illustrations on pp. 98–9)

Greater pectoral muscle

The pectoralis major has its origins in the clavicle, sternum, upper 4–6 rib cartilages and abdominal aponeurosis. It inserts to the crest of greater tubercle of the humerus. Its action is to draw the arm forward, adduct, and inwardly rotate it.

Pain may appear due to strain in weight lifting and throwing sports like javelin, cricket and racket sports. It is felt in the

With the arm abducted to stretch the belly of the pectoralis major muscle, the fingers strengthened by the other hand apply deep longitudinal stroking

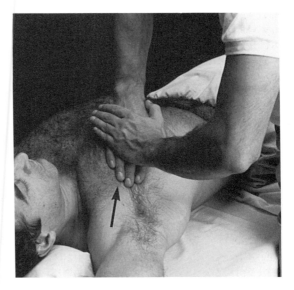

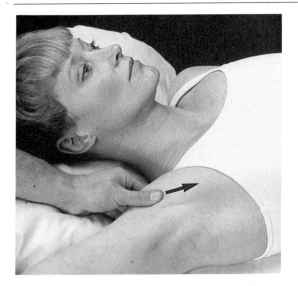

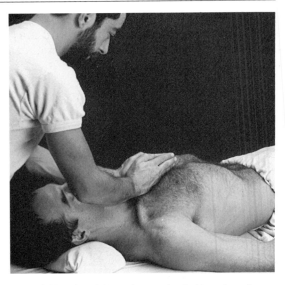

With the arm beside the head the attachment and lateral part of the pectoralis major muscle become more accessible and are treated by deep longitudinal stroking with the thumb. The other hand is used to hold the arm

The radial border of the palms apply stroking along the sternal muscle and outwards to the attachments of the great pectoral muscles. The palms of the hands, supporting each other, run along the sternum

chest, particularly when the shoulder is drawn backwards, and pain may also radiate to the shoulder. When occurring on the left side it may misleadingly simulate pain from coronary disease. Pain may also be referred to the breast, which may make women worry about breast cancer. This fear can be further strengthened as swelling and tenderness may appear due to blockages in the numerous lymphatic channels in the area due to compression of tense pectoral muscles. Examination by a medical practitioner should always be performed in these cases. The pectoralis major is a superficial muscle, and the cause of pain is easy to find through careful palpation. Stroking massage is an effective treatment.

Sternal muscle

This runs downwards along the sternum and is present in only five per cent of people and has no known function. However, it can sometimes cause severe chest pain

which may radiate to the shoulder. Even light massage gives considerable relief and it is easy to give self treatment.

Subclavius muscle

This muscle runs from the first rib laterally, attaching to the inferior surface of the clavicle and acting to protect the sternoclaviclar joint against excessive strain.

Deep friction applied using one finger strengthened by another on the subclavius muscle

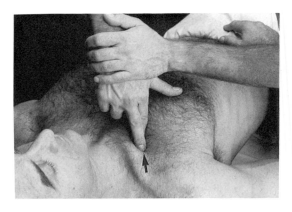

It is subject to trauma with similar activities to the pectoralis major and may also simulate coronary disease with chest pain radiating to the arm. Pain is most acutely felt when bringing the shoulder backwards. One should become familiar with its location by palpation, just below the clavicle and beneath the pectoralis muscle. Deep friction massage is effective treatment if applied in the correct place.

Smaller pectoral muscle

This lies beneath the major muscle running from ribs 3-5 and inserting into the coracoid process of the scapula. It draws the shoulders downwards and forwards. It also acts to lift the ribs upwards on inhalation (see the section on respiratory muscles in this chapter).

Strains usually occur in the upper part of the muscle in throwing sports like javelin and racket sports like tennis. Pain is felt mainly in the front of the shoulder and in the acromioclavicular joint, and is increased when the shoulder is moved both backwards and forwards. The source of pain may be difficult to locate as it is overlapped by the greater pectoral muscle, and other muscles in the area soon also beome stiff and tender. Diagnosis is thus often missed and emphasis is put on treating a totally different area. The brachial plexus may become compressed due to muscle tension near the insertion to the coracoid process causing entrapment symptoms (pain, numbness, tingling) in the arm. Shoulder pain easily tends to become chronic if treatment is not given at an early stage. Deep stroking and stretching are effective treatments when directly applied to the trauma. Massage of the whole area is necessary to treat secondary muscle tension and aching.

Serratus anterior muscle

This muscle has its origin in ribs 1-9 and attaches to the costal surface of the vertebral border of the scapula. It draws the scapula forward, abducts and rotates it, helping to raise the arm.

The serratus anterior may become overstrained in the same sports as mentioned above. The muscle attachments under the scapula hold it firmly against the chest

Deep transverse stroking applied with both thumbs to the pectoralis minor muscle. Special attention should be given to treatment of the upper part of it. The arm should be on the side of the trunk to ensure maximal relaxation of the pectoralis major muscle, allowing more effective treatment of the muscle beneath it

With the arm brought up beside the head to reveal the serratus anterior muscle, longitudinal stroking is applied along it, and along the course of ribs with the palmar surface of the thumb. Because this is a very tender area sharp pressure is avoided and contact is made with the whole hand

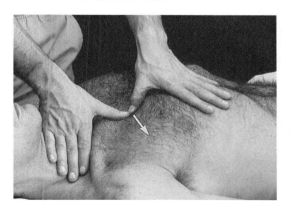

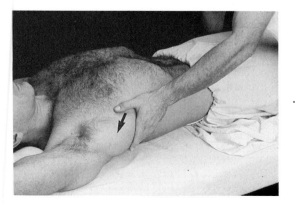

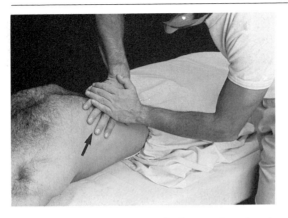

Deep stroking is applied using the fingers of one hand strengthened by the other hand, working between the ribs along the intercostal muscles

wall. Problems in the muscle may cause lateral chest pain, locally. The front part of the muscle can easily be reached with massage, but it is difficult to treat as it may be very tender and the area is also ticklish. The scapula lift is an effective way to stretch it.

PROBLEMS RELATING TO THE MUSCLES OF THE HEAD

Pain originating in the head muscles may not only be referred to other muscles but may also simulate painful conditions in different structures. These problems are at least as common in sportsmen as with non-active people. They are worth considering if any of the painful conditions listed below are present. Where no pathological cause is found, sometimes after many expensive examinations, the symptoms are often inappropriately thought to be psychogenic in origin. This is often due to poor, if any, examination of the muscles, and by not considering the causative effect of referred pain. With symptomatic treatment using painkillers the condition often returns when the effect of the drug wears off. This cannot be considered to be good treatment.

It is important to be aware of possible tension in the head muscles as effective treatment by massage can be applied and give good results.

Painful conditions, which may be caused by referred pain from muscles are:

Toothache
...masseter muscle; both upper and lower molar teeth
...temporal muscle; upper teeth
...digastric muscle; lower front teeth.

Eye pain (sometimes combined with blurred vision)
...temporalis muscle
...masseter muscle
...orbicularis oculi muscle

Chin pain (may simulate maxillary sinusitis, especially when having a cold)
...masseter muscle
...zygomatig muscle
...pterygoid muscle

Ear pain
...masseter muscle
...temporal muscle
...sternocleidomastoid muscle
...pterygoid muscles

Headache (frontal and occipital)
...occipito-frontalis (epicranius) muscles
...muscles attaching to occiput
...erector muscles of the spine
...sternocleidomastoid
Temporal
...temporal muscle
...masseter muscle

Throat ache (swallowing difficulties, 'tense voice')
...digastric muscle
...pterygoid muscles
...sternocleidomastoid muscles

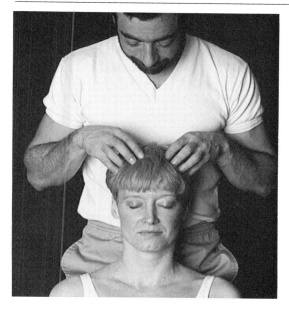
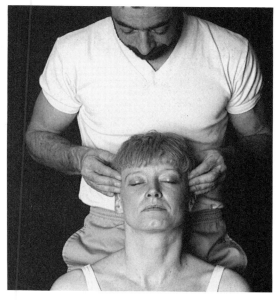

Above left: Pressure with small rotatory movements by the fingertips applied on the epicranial muscle and aponeurosis on the top of the head. The therapist starts from the front edge of the hairline and moves gradually backwards to the base of the skull. *Above right:* Pressure with small rotatory movements applied on the temporal muscle. The therapist starts from the midline of the forehead moving gradually backwards along both sides up to the back midline of the skull

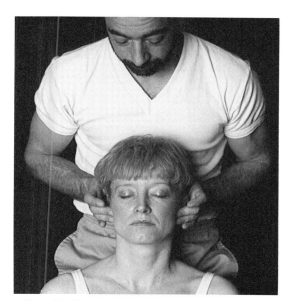
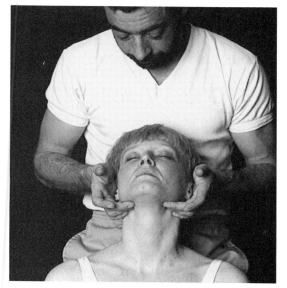

Above left: Pressure by the fingertips with small rotatory movements on the masseter muscle. *Above right:* Gentle stroking applied on the sublingual muscles starting from the chin and directed towards the neck.

ABDOMEN

The straight muscle of the abdomen

Rectus abdominus arises from ribs 5–7. It runs down the front of the abdomen inserting into the pubic crest. There is a tendinous band between the muscles on the right and left sides and there are three clearly felt transverse tendinous intersections and one smaller one near each end. They are often at slightly different heights on each side. The muscle is surrounded by fascia (rectus sheath).

Lateral abdominal muscles

The external oblique muscle arises from the outer surface of ribs 5–12 and runs diagonally forwards and downwards attaching to the rectus sheet and the iliac crest via a flat aponeurosis. The internal oblique muscle originates from thoracolumbar fascia, iliac crest and inguinal ligament. It fans out to insert into the lower border of the last three ribs and aponeurosis along the rectus sheath. The transverse muscle originates from the same area as the internal oblique muscle and internal surface of ribs 7–12 running to the rectus sheath.

These muscles flex and rotate the trunk and are the antagonists for the back muscles. They are the main muscles used in forced expiration. In sports requiring a big single effort, like powerlifting, the abdominal muscles are of primary importance, inducing pre-tension to the back muscles just before the lift and so stabilising the trunk. By holding the breath when lifting heavy weights, intra-abdominal and thoracic pressure increases and some of the load is mediated by these cavities to the pelvis, depending on the amount of forward bend also involved. More important, however, is the stabilisation of the trunk, as the back is vulnerable in side bending and rotary movements when bearing a heavy load.

Strains in the abdominal muscles most often affect the rectus abdominus near the attachment to the symphysis pubis. It is due to vigorous effort involving extension of the back and hip often combined with rotation. It often occurs in sports like skating, gymnastics, pole vault and from poor technique when using weights in strength training. Strains in the oblique muscles can occur with forceful rotatory movements like in javelin throwing and

The sportsman raises his neck and shoulders from the couch, so holding the abdomen muscles slightly contracted. The pads of the thumbs supporting each other are used to apply deep longitudinal stroking in sections to the rectus abdominus muscle

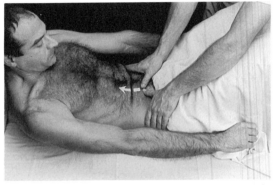

The fingers of one hand strengthened by the other hand are used to apply deep friction to the oblique muscles and to the lateral border of the rectus abdominis muscle

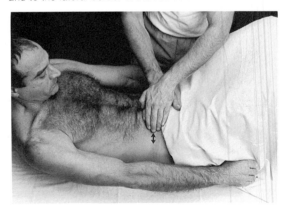

shot put. Excessive strain in the abdominal muscles can often lead to pain, which may simulate internal diseases. In the lower abdomen it could give similar symptoms to cystitis, urinary tract disorders or even appendicitis. In the upper abdomen it may be confused with gall stones and stomach pains. If the abdomen is palpated with the muscles relaxed the tender areas may stay unidentified and the cause of pain remain a mystery. When the muscle is contracted during examination pain can be easily located and treated by massage. Usually one can feel hard areas in the contracted muscle band, but there may be only trigger points which are tender. The muscle layer is not thick so it responds quickly to massage, and good results can often be obtained with just one treatment.

Abdominal massage is used frequently to induce general relaxation. This is because via the abdominal cavity one has close contact with the autonomous nervous system. This can be very useful in treating painful functional conditions in the abdomen, and gives relief with constipation and diarrhoea. Pre-competition stress can create painful symptoms in the abdomen and are fairly common with some sportsmen, resulting in poor performance. The symptoms may be eased by drugs, but abdominal muscle tension may still remain and restrict performance (see the following section on respiratory muscles). When abdomen massage is given to a sportsman, it should be done with the muscles both relaxed and with them in slight contraction, thus getting the greatest benefit for relieving local muscle tension as well as general stress (see the chapter on abdominal massage).

Iliopsoas muscle

This muscle runs from the back of the abdominal cavity from T12-L4 (psoas part) and iliac fossa (iliacus part) and attaches to the lesser trochanter of the femur. It is the strongest muscle in flexing the hip. It rotates the thigh medially and laterally depending on its position.

It is subject to strain in sports like weight lifting, hill running, jumping and hurdling. In 'sit-ups', after the shoulder blades are lifted from the floor and the abdominal muscles are contracted, the iliopsoas is the muscle that lifts the trunk up. In cases of prolapsed disc in the upper lumbar vertebrae the iliopsoas may go into protective spasm restricting all movement in the back. This spasm may affect just one side, thus causing rotation in the vertebrae, or on both sides causing a strong forward leaning posture. Spasm protects the nerve roots from being compressed more by the prolapsed disc.

Due to its location deep in the abdominal cavity it is a very difficult muscle to treat with massage, and only slight compression may be applied, which is not of practical importance in treatment. Muscle testing is the best way of identifying tension, and stretching (MET) should be applied for treatment.

RESPIRATORY MUSCLES

In all sports the respiratory muscles are an important factor in achieving good results. Endurance sportsmen must be able to keep them relaxed so that they can contract effectively and can be used economically to avoid exhaustion. In activities which require short burst at maximum effort, like in weight lifting, all the muscles need to contract simultaneously and be able to maintain this for several seconds against the load, and so increase pressure in the abdominal and thoracic cavities. The function of these muscles is even important in sports which do not require intensive muscle effort, such as shooting, where a smooth relaxed respiratory rhythm is needed.

Deep muscles

Superficial muscles

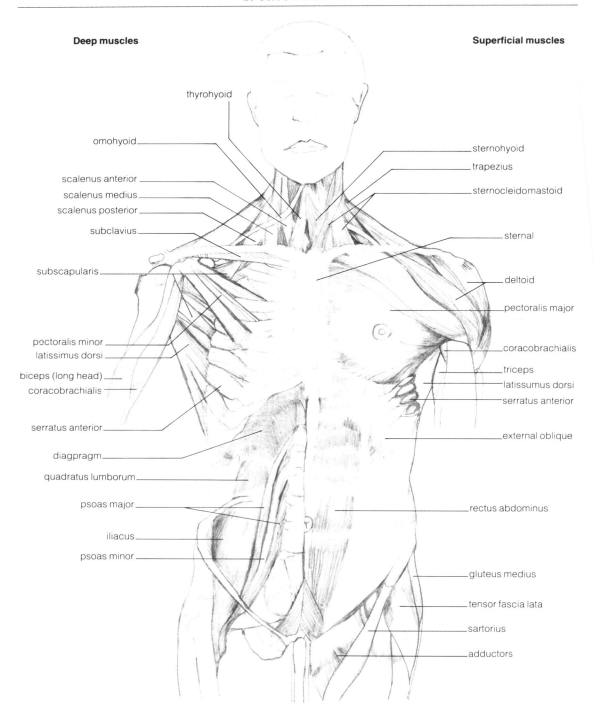

thyrohyoid

omohyoid

scalenus anterior

scalenus medius

scalenus posterior

subclavius

subscapularis

pectoralis minor

latissimus dorsi

biceps (long head)

coracobrachialis

serratus anterior

diagpragm

quadratus lumborum

psoas major

iliacus

psoas minor

sternohyoid

trapezius

sternocleidomastoid

sternal

deltoid

pectoralis major

coracobrachialis

triceps

latissumus dorsi

serratus anterior

external oblique

rectus abdominus

gluteus medius

tensor fascia lata

sartorius

adductors

13   Torso

Bones

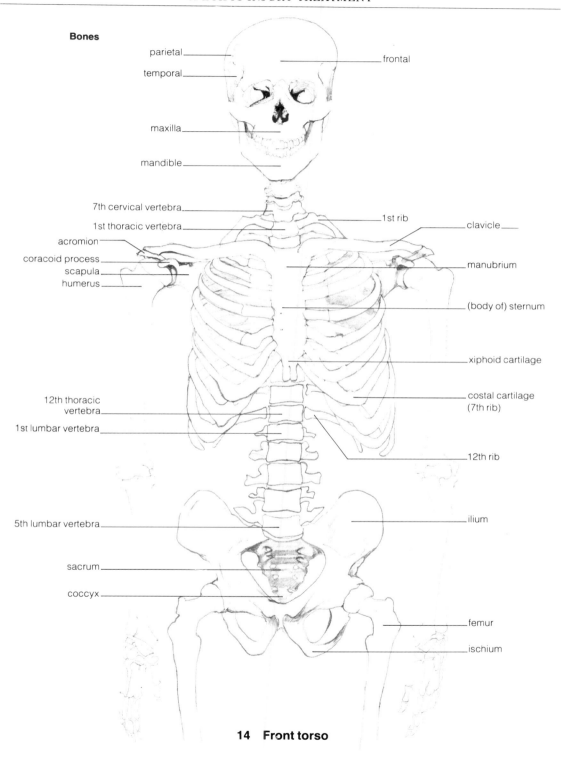

parietal

temporal

frontal

maxilla

mandible

7th cervical vertebra

1st thoracic vertebra

1st rib

clavicle

acromion

coracoid process

scapula

humerus

manubrium

(body of) sternum

xiphoid cartilage

12th thoracic vertebra

1st lumbar vertebra

costal cartilage (7th rib)

12th rib

5th lumbar vertebra

ilium

sacrum

coccyx

femur

ischium

14   Front torso

The respiratory rate and depth are controlled by the autonomous nervous system, but can also be controlled voluntarily. This is important in stress situations and, for example, after weight lifting where there is often a tendency to hyperventilate after increased effort. This leads to excessive deprivation of carbon dioxide from the blood and respiratory alkalosis, causing muscle tension and poor coordination. Proper use of the respiratory muscles is only possible with good posture. If there is a tendency to shrink forward (thoracic kyphosis) it is not possible to completely fill the lungs with fresh air. If the lower back tends to curve inwards (lumbar lordosis) it is not possible to effectively empty the lungs of air. These factors are very important, as good performance in endurance sports essentially depends on the effective removal of carbon dioxide from the blood when breathing out, and absorbtion of fresh oxygen to replace it when breathing in. When postural problems limit trunk rotation and sidebending both inspiration and expiration become restricted also. Although sportsmen are relatively fit, postural problems may affect them, particularly during periods of intensive training due to muscle tension and imbalance. Once identified, these can be improved through special individually tailored exercises and stretching as well as massage and mobilisation directed to the affected areas.

Diaphragm

This is an elevated dome shaped muscle arising from the vertebral bodies Th12–L3, ribs 7–12 and the sternum. In the centre is a clover-leaf shaped tendinous area through which the esophagus, aorta and vena cava pass. At rest respiration can be performed completely by the diaphragm. On inspiration the diaphragm muscle contracts, flattening the dome downwards. This creates a vacuum in the thoracic cavity which is filled by the expanding lungs drawing in air. When the lungs have been filled the diaphragm relaxes automatically and returns to its resting domed position increasing thoracic pressure and pushing the deoxygenated air out of the lungs.

Problems in the diaphragm muscle arise most often when a sportsman starts endurance training which he is not used to, or after a long lay off. Difficulties may appear also in competition with extreme effort. This will appear as abdominal pain, which is felt usually on the right side of the navel and is a result of excessive tension in the diaphragm. This is not a dangerous condition, but pain may become so intense that it is not possible to continue exercise. If the pain is not too severe one can try to release it via the reflexes. The sportsman may apply deep pressure sharply with thumb or fingers over the most tender area, or if that is not clear one should press the point in the lateral border of rectus abdominis muscle on the same level as the

With the sportsman's abdomen in a fully relaxed position: knees flexed, hands lying on the side and head resting on a cushion. The fingers of both hands are used to reach under the front lower arch of the thoracic cage. The sportsman is asked to breath in and out slowly and at the end of the outbreath the stretch is applied. The therapist widens the chest, applies a stretch to the upper part of the abdominal muscles and introduces pressure on the diaphragm near its attachments

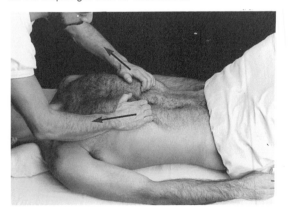

navel for ten to twenty seconds. This can be repeated a couple of times. If the pain is too severe to continue, the sportsman should lie down on his back and bend the knees to relax the abdomen muscles fully. Pressure release technique should be applied by pressing the fingers under the right and left arcus (ribs 7–9), at the same time breathing slowly and deeply in and out a few times. This gives a stretching effect on the diaphragm muscle which may relieve the pain and enable exercise to continue. The diaphragm muscle cannot be treated by massage, but the front attachments can be reached during abdominal massage.

Accessory respiratory muscles

Forced inspiration
upper and middle trapezius muscles elevate shoulders and draw them backwards
rhomboid muscles pull shoulders backwards
levator scapulae muscles elevate shoulders
scalenus muscles elevate the thorax
sternocleidomestoid muscles elevate thorax
pectoralis minor widens and elevates the chest
serratus posterior superior draws ribs 2–5 backwards
serratus posterior inferior draws ribs 9–12 backwards
intercostal muscles draw ribs together

Forced expiration
straight, oblique and transverse muscles of the abdomen increase intra-abdominal pressure and draw thorax downwards
pectoralis major muscles pull shoulders forward
serratus anterior muscles pull shoulder-blades forward
quadratus lumborum muscle lowers the ribcage.

During intensive physical exercise it is necessary for all the accessory inspiration muscles to work simultaneously, and a single lesion in one muscle can restrict the total breathing pattern. The importance of the accessory expiration muscles is also their function as antagonists to the inspiration muscles. Greater tension in these means more effort is needed on inspiration.

Both expiratory and inspiratory muscles contract at the same time during strong effort, like in weight-lifting, as the thoracic and intra-abdominal pressure is used to stabilise the back and also to carry some of the load. Strength and good function in these muscles is as important as in the muscles of the arms and legs.

When a sportsman finds that his performance seems to be below par, even though his training has been going well and there seem to be no problems in the muscles specifically related to his sport, one should consider treating the respiratory muscles. With endurance sportsmen it is important to treat these muscles on a regular basis. The frequency should be determined individually according to the degree of tension found.

Sharp pain felt in the chest or upper back during deep respiration is most often vertebrogenic in origin and is due to tension in the deep muscles of the back, which has been dealt with before in this chapter. Good function of the intervertebral joints and muscles of the back is necessary to normal respiration as the spine straightens during inspiration and becomes more curved during expiration. Muscle tension can frequently be released with massage and stretching, but there is also often restricted movement locally between a few vertebrae and manipulation may be required.

10
CONTRAINDICATIONS OF MASSAGE

Acute traumas
   open wounds
   muscle ruptures
   tendon ruptures
   contusions
   burns
   chilblains
   broken bones
Periostitis
Rheumatoid arthritis and gout
Bursitis
Myositis ossificans
Infections:
   bacterial
   viral
   fungal
Thrombosis
Artificial blood vessels
Bleeding disorders
Tumours

Many of the contraindications listed above are perhaps obvious, but there are times when there arises the question of whether one can safely treat a particular condition. Many of the conditions listed above will normally affect just one part or area of the body. Massage should not be applied to these areas, but it is often beneficial to treat the area around it as well as the body as a whole to improve circulation. There are also conditions where massage is totally prohibited. It is necessary to include in the list some conditions, which may not at first seem relevant to sports. Today sport for the handicapped is becoming increasingly popular, and there is lot of competition at very high standards. This adds a new dimension to sports therapy. It requires much more knowledge from the therapist to be able to take account of new problems which this brings about.

ACUTE TRAUMA

With treatment of acute traumas, refer to the relevant chapter in this book. It is clear that one cannot massage these acute conditions at the earliest stage, but the question is, when can such treatment begin? In the case of open wounds one has to wait for the scar to form (one to two weeks depending on, for example, the severity and area of the injury). Massage can only take place at such an early stage if extreme care is taken. One should work gently around the scar but not directly on it. The direction of the strokes must be towards the scar rather than away from it. This will prevent stretching the scar tissue which would induce more of it to form. One should not apply oil directly to the scar as it will make it softer and also induce excessive scar tissue formation in the skin. This cautious approach should be kept up until the scar has completely healed (often several months) which can be identified when the scar and surrounding tissue are the same colour. This approach should also be applied in cases of burns, chilblains or frostbite.

It is vital that massage treatment is used as soon after acute connective tissue trauma as is practically possible. This is to prevent the formation of scar tissue, adhesions and myositis ossificans and so promote the restoration of normal function. It is safe to give gentle treatment as soon as there is no risk of inducing new bleeding. This is dealt with in the chapter on the treatment of acute injuries. In most cases of broken bones immobilisation is vital for the healing process which makes the use of massage impossible. After the caste has been removed it is most often advisable to start the treatment immediately.

PERIOSTITIS

This is the inflammation of the connective tissue layer which covers the bone. It is often due to direct impact trauma causing bleeding under the periosteum or long-standing inflammation. In long term cases it may be verified by X-ray, because the area will have a tendency to calcify. Massage applied locally on it may cause irritation.

Tenoperiostitis is inflammation between the tendon and its attachment to the periosteum of the bone. It builds up gradually as a result of long-standing stress, although there may not be any painful warning signs. There is usually excessive muscle tension for a period leading up to the onset of tenoperiostitis. If this tension is removed by massage, at an early stage one may be able to prevent the condition from following, for example 'tennis elbow'. Massage can be applied also to remove scar tissue from the common tendon of extensor muscles and tendon of supinator muscle. When the periosteal inflammation has already developed over a long period of time and there has formed some calcification, local massage to the tendon attachment will cause pain and aggravate inflammation.

RHEUMATOID ARTHRITIS AND GOUT

These are inflammatory conditions which involve disturbances in the body's own defence mechanisms. They may involve one or several joints and the soft tissues around them. Symptoms of acute inflammation are: heat, swelling, redness, aching and stiffness. Massage is beneficial in soft tissue disorders when applied in the non-acute stage, but in acute states it may cause severe irritation and increased pain. Although acute inflammation may seem to be restricted to one joint, massaging other areas, especially if applying pressure to the periosteum, one may cause new local inflammation.

BURSITIS

A bursa is a sack containing a small amount of fluid and is positioned between different tissues near joints. The purpose of the bursa is to reduce friction between tissue layers during joint movement. Inflammation is caused by repeated pressure or excessive friction and is usually non-bacterial. The symptoms are: swelling, redness, heat, pain and tenderness which causes dysfunction.

Massage is always contraindicated when there appear major signs of inflammation like heat and redness as it will aggravate the condition. Cases of this sort should be referred to a medical practitioner. When the only symptoms are pain and/or swelling over the bursa, and no other signs of inflammation exist, it is beneficial to apply massage. One should use gentle deep friction to the tendon and muscle, working in a lateral direction to the way they lie. This will break down adhesions, loosen connective tissue and improve local circulation.

MYOSITIS OSSIFICANS

This is a rare process of ossification in a traumatised area of the muscle. Contusion or rupture of the muscles will often cause bleeding (haematoma) within or between them. If this blood is retained there it may become calcified. In the beginning there will be acute trauma symptoms and sometimes excessive bleeding, causing much swelling. Later on there may only be pain on exercise and diffused aching afterwards. Muscular activity and massage will aggravate the symptoms and lengthen the calcification process. The best treatment will usually be surgical.

Myositis ossificans is a condition which takes a long time to develop, and it prevents normal training. The best approach is a preventative one. Massive haemorrhage should be removed surgically at a very early stage before calcification begins. Smaller haemorrhage will benefit from massage treatment which will improve circulation and resorbtion of the haemorrhage.

INFECTIONS

There are two main reasons why one should be careful when dealing with infections. It is possible that the therapist may spread the infection to other areas of the body, and if it is a transmitable infection the therapist can of course catch it himself. People may feel pain without realising it is due to a recently developed infectious condition, so one must be aware of such possibilities. Some examples of the most common soft tissue infections affecting sportsmen are discussed below.

Bacterial Infections

Folliculitis can be caused by skin friction, and it is important to use enough oil to avoid it. It is usually only a mild infection of the hair follicle and will recover without treatment or by local anti-bacterial salve, which can be obtained from chemists without prescription. The skin areas affected by this condition should not be irritated by massage.

Lymphangitis usually originates from abrasions or small cuts in the hands or feet, where bacteria can invade lymphatic channels and be transported to tissues. One notices a red line running up the limb with tenderness as a first sign. If not treated in time there will appear local heat, swelling of the nearest lymph nodes, and fever.

Cellulitis is a bacterial infection in subcutaneous fat layers. It can appear anywhere in the body, causing local heat, redness, some swelling and pain. It may appear due to spreading of local folliculitis or abrasion.

Erysipelas can be a result of exceptionally long sustained exercise, for example long distance skiing and running. This will put excessive strain also on the body's immune system and its resistance drops temporarily. Increased muscle tension will cause stagnation of body fluids after exercise in the lower extremities. Friction at the epidermal layer caused by the exercise leads to a potential risk of bacteria entering the body. The symptoms will be fever, redness, swelling, heat and pain in the local area. To prevent it sportsmen should maintain good hygiene and try to normalise circulation to the legs as soon as possible by stretching and massage. The worst thing to do is to rest completely without any exercise. The treatment for bacterial infection should be sought from a medical practitioner. They are easily cured with antibiotics, and rest is essential until total recovery has taken place. Massage is prohibited until that time.

Viral infections

Influenza is the most common disease to affect sportsmen, occuring once or twice a year on average. Treatment is rest, and massage is contraindicated as long as the following general symptoms of infection exist: fever, fatigue and general aching. This is also the case when these symptoms exist with other conditions.

Viral infections affecting the skin are quite common in childhood (measles, chicken pox, rubella) but are rare among adults who have developed immunity through having already had the disease. In the early or mild cases there may only be a skin rash, and other common infectious symptoms are not present. These are droplet infections and are thus easily transmitted.

Herpes, which occurs in the mucous membrane of the mouth and genital area, cannot be transmitted through massage. There are other types of herpes where a group of small blisters occur on normal body skin which can be transmitted to the therapist through massage. Blisters on the skin which contain clear liquid are contraindication to massage. If there is any doubt, medical opinion should be sought.

Warts (verruca) are caused by viral infection of the skin. They are more common among young people, usually occurring on the hands and feet. Warts are benign growths in the skin. The masseur should avoid giving treatment over the area where they exist, because they may be transmitted.

Fungal infection

Ringworm is usually the result of poor hygiene and affects warm moist areas such as armpits, below the breasts, inguinal area and most commonly between the toes. It is often transmitted when using communal bathing facilities. It can be avoided by the sportsman wearing slippers in the shower, drying oneself carefully and using anti-perspirants rather than deodorants. Areas affected by ringworm appear red with white flakey skin and a characteristic odour. Treatment is a medication given locally as cream or powder. Massage should not be given over these areas as it will cause irritation. It does not transmit to the masseur if the skin of his hands are healthy and are washed after the treatment.

Another type of ringworm can establish itself under the nails and is also common among sportsmen. There is discolouration of the nail and white debris forms underneath it. Treatment is extraction of the nail and medication. This condition can be transmitted to the masseur if he treats an infected foot. Either avoid treatment in such cases or wash hands thoroughly afterwards and keep fingernails cut very short.

THROMBOSIS

Venous thrombosis is a clot of blood which stops the circulation in the vein. This is a condition which is very rare among sportsmen because it usually affects inactive people. It can, however, be a further complication during immobilisation after a sports trauma. Symptoms of venous thrombosis are local pain and sometimes also swelling and blue discolouration.

Phlebitis is a condition usually affecting varicose veins and is sometimes started by local trauma. Inflammation can even lead to circulatory block of the vein. Symptoms are very localised pain, tenderness and swelling; heat and redness are also noticed when phlebitis is superficial.

Both venous thrombosis and phlebitis require medical attention for accurate diagnosis and treatment. If there is a possibility of a thrombosis, massage treatment should not be given, as it can release the blood clot into the general circulation and cause thrombosis in other organs. If the sportsman reports sudden pain which appeared in the leg while at rest and with no obvious cause the therapist should consider the possibility of thrombosis.

ARTIFICIAL BLOOD VESSELS

Parts which have been implanted in the soft tissue, such as artificial blood vessels, should not be massaged over. Massage can cause irritation between normal and implanted tisssue and may sometimes even cause direct damage. Massage can, however, be safely applied over artificial joints.

BLEEDING DISORDERS

People suffering from bleeding disorders like haemophilia can receive only light relaxing massage. One should never apply deep massage because there is a danger of creating a haemorrhage in deep lying muscle tissue.

TUMOURS

While giving massage, the therapist makes a proper examination of the soft tissues which is rarely done by any other diagnostic or therapeutical method.

Most lumps found in the subcutaneous layer are made up of fat tissue. They have a typical consistency: the fat nodules are soft, freely movable against deeper tissues and are surrounded by a smooth capsule. Lumps found in muscle are usually made up of contracted muscle fibres. Local muscle nodules are hard and with a typical striated feel to them. With a little experience these are easy to identify.

Therapists should be aware of the possibility of malignant tumours which can appear in the skin, subcutaneously, in the muscles and underlying bones. The history of the complaint can be misleading. For example, the sportsman may report that he occasionally experiences intense pain when using high effort. One naturally thinks at first that it is a soft tissue injury.

The therapist should palpate a lump carefully, and if it does not feel like the type of benign lump described above and experienced before then medical advice should always be sought. If intensive massage treatment is applied to malignant tissue there is a risk of irritation which can speed the growth and even spread the malignancy.

11
CORRECT USE OF SPORTS MASSAGE

Massage is a highly technical skill which can only be acquired with much practice. One has to be able to work without getting exhausted and also avoid doing it the wrong way. There are many mistakes that can be made by the therapist who is not experienced in treating sportsmen. Below we give advice which one should study carefully to avoid mistakes.

TIMING

It is a mistake to give a sportsman his first massage just before a competition. Strong deep massage induces a high level of relaxation which may hinder the sportsman's ability to reach top performance. All people respond in different ways to massage, and so they should get experience during a normal training period to discover their own requirements. If the sportsman is receiving regular massage he will often prefer a lighter massage a couple of days before competing, and it is also necessary sometimes to deal with local traumas just before. Massage treatment should be less relaxing and more stimulating before competition. Effective deep massage should be applied at least a week before an event to allow time for the full benefits to be felt.

After hard training sessions and competition is the best time for massage, before muscle sensitivity and stiffness set in. At this stage the massage will be more comfortable and effective than if there is a long delay, and it will also be easier for the therapist. If the sportsman has to wait several hours he should try to keep the muscles warm and keep moving. If massage cannot be done the same day one should aim to have it the day after.

FREQUENCY

Tissues need time to recover from massage so the full effects can be seen. Recovery can take normally from one to three days, but with some very sensitive people it may take up to a week. If the interval between sessions is too long the condition which may have improved could slip back and the therapist has to start again at the beginning. This is particularly important when training is continued between treatments.

When serious training is leading towards peak performance the sportsman should discuss and plan with his trainer and masseur how massage sessions should be fitted in to his training schedule. During periods of intensive training early in the season, when the sportsman is building up basic strength and fitness, massage should be given more frequently. This is a hard period of training, and it is important to let the tissues recover totally as quickly as possible and especially to ensure there are no areas of excessive tension which could lead to serious injury.

Ideally the sportsman should have massage daily, or at least after every hard training session. This is standard practice for top sportsmen in many Eastern European countries, but for economical and practical reasons it is not common in the West. The competitive sportsman should consider having massage at least once a week. Ideally this should be done after the hardest training session of the week. Massage should always be followed by one or two days of lighter training, which should be the case anyway after hard training. When massage is given only once a week it is important to make it deep and thorough, whereas if done more often it should be lighter, and the parts treated can be varied according to the particular needs. Even with very hard training it is possible to give an overdose of massage if it is applied almost daily with maximal effort. This will lead to excessive muscle relaxation and difficulties in performing training at a high level.

Amateur or recreational sportsmen who train regularly but may not push themselves to maximum limits should also consider the use of massage to prevent injury at least twice a month. Many amateurs push themselves regularly to their maximum effort and actually go through more stress than the top sportsmen because they do not have the same conditioning and may also have occupational stress to cope with. These people should consider having massage more regularly because they may be at even greater risk of overtraining and traumas.

DURATION OF TREATMENT

The normal duration of a full body massage should be between one and one-and-a-half hours, and a half body massage between one-half and three-quarter hours. It is not practical to try to divide this into set times for individual parts of the body because the condition of the soft tissue will be different in every sportsman. The therapist often finds areas that require special attention which also have to be dealt with during the time alloted for the whole session. Ability to divide the time between different parts develops quickly with practice.

It does take at least one hour to give a thorough full body sports massage, and it is not a good practice to try to squeeze it into less. If one is short of time it is better to give a half body massage or just concentrate on the most important areas. Over recent years it has become popular to use electro and heat therapies as initial treatments, which may take up half of the session time. This has led to an unfortunate reduction of time given to massage, as the total therapy time has remained the same. It is impossible to give massage with the same effect when so little time is devoted to it. This will lead to an increase in the number of sessions required, and even then the results may be poor. Electro and heat therapies are very different from massage and should not be considered as equal alternatives, although they may often be good as additional treatments.

PRESSURE AND EFFORT

There is no standard for the amount of pressure one puts into the massage. Every sportsman and even each massage will have different requirements depending on the body type, muscle composition, the training cycle, the sport, and of course any actual problems the sportsman may have.

If one compares an endurance sportsman with one who uses short bursts of high effort (e.g. sprinters, weight lifters, wrestlers) very different body and muscle types will be found for the two. In the power sports, athletes have muscles which have a larger proportion of fast twitch fibres and the muscles are bigger with more natural tension. In endurance sports they have a higher proportion of slow twitch fibres and the muscles are smaller, softer and more relaxed. This difference can be quite extreme; for example, the quadriceps muscle may consist of ninety per cent fast twitch fibres in the sprinter compared with a marathon runner who may have ninety per cent slow twitch fibres.

When giving massage to these two types of people there are important differences. The power sportsman will require more effort to reach deeper layers of muscles. One should aim to restore the level of tension natural to the muscle and not try to achieve the same softness as with the endurance sportsman. In sports requiring fast performance and reaction times, too high a level of relaxation will have a negative effect on performance.

The endurance sportsman benefits from a high level of relaxation to ensure good circulation over a long period of exercise and to speed up recovery. Less tension also enables muscles to move more freely and efficiently resulting in better performance. Massage in this case should be aimed more at relaxation and softening the muscles.

Unfortunately few sports fall neatly into these two categories. Sports like football, basketball, tennis and boxing have matches which last a long time and require endurance. On the other hand, the sportsman has to perform many short bursts of high effort and needs fast reaction times. Here the muscle type of the sportsman will be more mixed between slow and fast twitch fibres. The therapist must become familiar with the different sports as well as each individual sportsman and adapt the massage accordingly. It is therefore not good for the sportsman to change his therapist often.

BALANCED TREATMENT

In many sports, like racket sports, javelin and shot put, one side of the body is trained harder and becomes more developed. This will create an imbalance, as the muscles on one side are not only bigger but also more tense, which will create postural stress. This problem is often taken into account in training programmes by exercising the weaker side as well. Therapists should also consider this problem and work to equalise tension on both sides. This is done by working more intensely for a longer time on the side with excessive tension.

In sports requiring equal effort from both sides of the body, like running, weight lifting and swimming, the stress from training will be equal on both sides. Trauma or injury, however, will usually only affect one side, creating an imbalance because of pain and dysfunction. While effectively treating the traumatised side and restoring its proper function, it is possible to make it more efficient and stronger than the other side. If the therapist does not treat the non-traumatised side at all one may create a severe imbalance leading to a risk of traumatising the previously healthy side. For example, a weight lifter, who received treatment to the left triceps muscle due to strain, in the next training session may strain the right triceps tendon while doing heavy bench press.

Imbalance may also exist in antagonist muscles. For example, a sprinter who received treatment for cramp in the quadriceps muscle was recovering well from that, but at the next hard effort he strained the hamstring of the same leg. This was due to excessive tension in the whole thigh, but treatment was only given to the front side, leaving the hamstrings vulnerable to injury. So, even when treating a specific problem, it is essential to treat the opposing muscles as well.

The therapist should *always* ensure that the treatment is balanced. The sportsman should be treated as a whole and not only concentrating on specific injury problems.

POSITIONING

It has been a long-standing tradition to use the prone and supine as standard treatment positions for massage treatment.

109

Normally these are indeed the best positions for giving maximum relaxation, but this is not necessarily the case in some conditions. When treating acute back traumas, for example, the patient may feel considerable pain or discomfort in these positions. This will not only reduce the benefits of the treatment but may make the condition even worse. If muscles remain contracted for a long time in a bad position they will be difficult to release.

With acute conditions of this kind the therapist should ask the patient to lie in a position which gives maximum comfort. This will probably be half side lying, but in cases of acute neck and shoulder conditions the sitting position may be preferred. Pillows can be used to give support if necessary. The comfort of the patient should be checked several times, especially if the treatment takes a long time, and the position should be changed if necessary.

12
TREATMENT OF ACUTE INJURIES

When a sportsman suffers an acute musculoskeletal injury at a sporting venue it should be a medical practitioner or therapist who is specialised in sports injuries, and has the proper equipment, who gives the initial treatment. For most acute injuries the treatment given is fairly similar (RICE: rest, ice, compression and elevation).

REST

With any acute trauma injury the first thing to do is to rest the affected part. Activity may increase bleeding, inflammation and induce more swelling. The movement may cause further tearing of soft tissue so one should not continue exercising, even though with effective early treatment the symptoms may not be apparent. To allow proper rest it may be necessary to use strapping, slings, castes, collars, corsets or crutches.

ICE

Cold applied locally to the site of the injury or muscle cramp is an effective measure against pain as it reduces conductivity in the nerves and chills pain receptors. It slows blood circulation and stops bleeding. Cold will stop the inflammatory process and prevent the swelling from effusion. It will also help release muscle spasm.

Where the injury affects the tissue near the surface or at the lower arms or lower legs, cold should be applied for only ten minutes at a time. With deep injuries cold can be applied for up to twenty minutes.

The treatment can be repeated when the part starts to warm up again, which will depend on body and surrounding temperature. One may continue with cold therapy for one to two days following the injury.

Cold therapy should always be restricted to the local injury area only. If it is applied to a large area it may cause a strong reflex, opening the blood vessels and increasing the circulation after a short period of time. This will make the whole initial treatment ineffective. The same will happen if the cold pack is removed too early; this is a common fault with using cold sprays applied for some minutes.

Cold sprays are popular because they are easy to carry. One should avoid the use of cold sprays on acute traumas because it is practically impossible to effectively cool the deep tissue without causing the skin to freeze. If using cold sprays one should have a routine method of application including spraying times with set intervals in between, as recommended by the manufacturer. It is safer and far more effective to use an ice pack wrapped in a wet towel or iced water. It is also possible to apply compression at the same time when using ice packs .

COMPRESSION

Compression should be applied to stop bleeding and prevent swelling. One should not just wrap the traumatised area as this will spread the pressure, and if wrapping is applied to a limb it will restrict blood flow to the extremity. This can be avoided by using a hard pad on the injury site and putting the wrapping around it so the pressure is concentrated. If ice is not immediately available, one should apply compression as a first treatment.

ELEVATION

The injured part should be kept in an elevated position whenever possible. This is to prevent the pressure caused by gravity leading to local swelling around the trauma and distal to it in the extremities.

The result of giving good acute treatment is effective pain relief. By preventing swelling and inflammatory processes which cause further tissue damage, RICE treatment will help start the healing process early. It will also minimise a risk of forming chronic problems like scar tissue and adhesions, which can restrict movement.

When the injured sportsman is moved to home or a medical centre the injured part should be kept immobile and not be allowed to bear weight. Good treatment immediately following the trauma will leave no obvious sign of the injury, even though there might be a massive trauma like a total ligament rupture. In the field of sports it is important to consider the severity of the trauma and not be fooled by what may appear to be a miraculous recovery.

POST ACUTE TREATMENT

Rest recommended as a post acute treatment does not always mean bed rest. Usually it means avoiding weight bearing and resistant type movements. Passive movements and isometric exercises are important to start at a fairly early stage depending on the trauma and medical advice. This is to prevent atrophy of muscles and tendons, adhesions, ligament and joint capsule contraction.

Massage, ultrasound, heat treatments and passive exercises can usually be applied two or three days after an acute soft tissue injury, when the risk of swelling and bleeding has decreased. The purpose of post acute treatment is to speed up the healing process and to prevent the complications described above.

Heat treatment is commonly recommended in post acute injuries as well as for general aches and pains, but the proper use of it is often not explained, which may lead to poor results. Heat should not be applied for more than half an hour at a time as tissue metabolism begins to suffer if a high temperature is maintained for too long. Treatment can be repeated soon after the temperature of the tissues has returned to normal. The use of hot and cold in combination can also be very effective. Alternating between hot and cold every one minute increases circulation and also gives increased stimulation to the autonomic nervous system.

Gentle superficial stroking massage can be applied to strains two or three days after the injury, and usually with mild and moderate strains deep stroking and friction techniques can be started after seven days as fibrous tissue has started to form. The treatment should always be applied without causing pain, which will ensure that no further tissue damage is caused by massage. With severe strains medical advice and control should be sought before starting the treatment.

For the competitive sportsman the time missed from training whilst recovery from the trauma will have an adverse effect on performance. Every day lost from training due to rest after the trauma will cause a drop in sporting ability. But it is important that the sportsman does not panic and commence training before advised to, which may cause chronic conditions and have far more detrimental effect on performance.

Rest alone does not always ensure full and speedy recovery for injuries.

13
ADVICE AND INFORMATION

Sports massage should be regarded as a therapy which goes beyond the treatment given on the couch. The hands of the experienced masseur are a good diagnostic tool which can examine the condition of the muscles thoroughly in a way which is not done in any other therapy. The information received can be used by the sportsman and coach so they can improve training schedules and take measures to avoid overuse and future injuries.

STRETCHING

Where the therapist finds excessive muscle tension, the sportsman should be advised to stretch that part effectively. This will continue the benefits of the treatment and help him improve his general conditioning over the long term. Stretching will reduce muscle tension and so prevent the development of overuse injuries.

Where muscle tension is contributing to a specific injury, advice on stretching is even more important. The sportsman can treat his own injury many times a day by stretching the right part. This will not only speed the healing process but often has positive psychological effects as he feels more in control of the problem and he can monitor his own progress.

Sporting performance benefits greatly from the improved flexibility which comes from stretching. A muscle has to work harder and use more energy to move a joint if the muscle opposing that movement is too tense. With greater flexibility movement becomes more efficient so performance and technique can improve.

All sportsmen should have a stretching programme which they carry out regularly. How to stretch properly is just as important as the positions themselves, and advice on both may be necessary. Unfortunately many sportsmen today develop their stretching programme from a variety of sources, not all of which may be good. It is important to advise the sportsman on a stretching routine which can be carried out correctly and according to his individual needs and the demands of his sport.

MUSCLE BALANCE

The most common aim in sports massage is to reduce excessive muscle tension as this is a typical cause of injury problems. Muscle weakness is another important factor to consider. A weak muscle obviously becomes fatigued quicker and so is more likely to become strained. A problem for some sportsmen occurs when there is weakness in a part of a muscle or muscle group creating an imbalance in the system as a whole. This may cause local muscle strain or pain in the joint, but other consequences can be more serious. The sportsman may continue hard training unaware of the gradual build-up of fatigue and tension in a small area and unwittingly make compensations for it by changing technique. This can lead to a variety of other potentially more serious problems.

The strength of a muscle can be approximately judged by its size, though the amount of tension has a significant effect also. Imbalance can exist between the same muscles on different sides of the body. This can often actually be seen, and an experienced therapist can tell that there is an imbalance by feeling the muscles on both sides simultaneously.

These observations can usually be tested by using active or resisted movements. The dynamic strength of a muscle can be judged by getting the sportsman to use it to move the joint against a force such as gravity, or, for strong muscles, some weight or other resistance. In cases where there is restricted joint movement, or trauma in other muscles in the area, isometric exercises can be used. These involve the sportsman contracting the muscle without moving the joint. Any differences found between the two sides of the body will be felt by the therapist when he resists these movements. Frequent testing not only makes the sportsman aware of any problems, but also gives him a way of monitoring progress in restoring balance, and demonstrates which exercises can be used to do this. If pain is experienced when doing these exercises it is a sign that there is a problem other than weakness to be diagnosed.

Imbalance can exist between muscles which oppose each other in the movement of a joint and can affect both sides of the body equally. Due to the complex arrangement of muscle groups, the way the body moves and the force of gravity, opposing muscles do not require equal strength. For example, the hamstrings are smaller than the quadriceps. Accurate measurement of muscle strength is difficult and requires clinical testing procedures, but with experience and using basic testing methods it is possible to make a fairly accurate, though intuitive, assessment.

Massage does not directly improve muscle strength. A muscle may feel stronger to the sportsman after treatment but this is due to improved efficiency through the effects of massage. The therapist can only advise on the situation and recommend strengthening exercises. Isometric exercises can be included easily into a stretching programme. Advice on weight training or using an alternative sport or exercise should be given when there is a difference in dynamic strength.

OVERTRAINING

Too many sportsmen today continue training with a chronic injury until it becomes worse and forces them to stop. Sports massage helps to identify tissue damage, the sportsman will become more aware of it, and so take appropriate measures. It is often necessary to advise a sportsman to cut down on training to allow time for proper recovery. There are times when this will cause conflict with the sportsman's goals and determination, but the consequences of excessive training and increased risk of injury should be emphasised.

Many amateur and recreational sportsmen train to a high level but do not have the back-up of coaches and trainers to advise them. They can benefit from a therapist's advice on the condition of the muscles to help monitor and plan their training programme and prevent the dangers of overtraining.

For a sports club or team the therapist can play a special role. For practical reasons teams do much of their training together following the same programme. But not all sportsmen will necessarily respond in the same way, even though their performance standards may be similar. The masseur will see the relative differences among the sportsmen and see how they are responding to training. This may help the trainer make adjustments in their programme.

SELF TREATMENT

For practical or financial reasons it may not be possible for a sportsman to come for treatment as often as necessary. One should give advice on self treatment using ice and/or heat with traumas. Where scar tissue or adhesions are present the therapist can demonstrate to the sportsman how to apply deep friction to the affected area. Advice on self treatment is often easier to explain whilst giving the treatment as the exact location of treatment is identified.

GENERAL ADVICE

It is always important to try to find the cause of an injury so it may be prevented from happening again. The number of possible causes of sports injury is infinite so the therapist needs to keep an open mind when giving advice. Throughout this book references are made to the main causes of injury, like overtraining, where giving advice can be quite straightforward. But sometimes the cause of injury can be rather obscure. For example, a runner may do all his training along the same side of a road which has a camber. This will cause repeated stress on one side of the body which can lead to injury. Track runners who train in the same direction round the track all the time risk a similar fate.

To be able to give good advice it is necessary to know a great deal about the sportsman's training methods. It is helpful to discuss them during treatment. Much becomes apparent through the massage; for example, if one finds tension in a localised area, the therapist should ask if a particular stretch for that part is being included in the stretching routine. If it is not he can be shown how to do so at the end of the session. If it is, then one should check that it is being carried out correctly. If there is an overuse injury, the therapist should ask detailed questions about train-ing methods used, to try to find the particular aspect which is creating the problem.

PSYCHOLOGICAL ATTITUDE

The therapist who gives sports massage has a unique relationship with the sportsman. Although the purpose of sports massage is primarily a physical one, the psychological effect of receiving massage should not be ignored. For the time the sportsman is being treated he is in a warm, comfortable room without any disturbances, enjoying the very pleasant sensation of being massaged. For some sportsmen this is a welcome opportunity for quiet, deep relaxation, and the therapist should be aware of this and not indulge in unnecessary conversation. But for others it may be an opportunity to talk, not just about sport, but often about other factors which may affect their lives. Problems affecting the private life of a sportsman have an affect on performance, and the masseur often seems to be the one in the middle who they can talk to. One should not instigate this type of conversation, but if it does arise it should not be discouraged. A therapist needs to be a sympathetic listener and keep such conversations confidential.

OTHER TREATMENTS

Massage is a very effective therapy, but there will always be conditions which do not respond to treatment. Spinal joint problems are often relieved by massage of the surrounding muscles, and spontaneous recovery can occur when good relaxation has been obtained. However, if no significant relief is achieved after two or three treatments, one should not carry on in the hope that something may eventually happen. Medical advice should be sought, and if there is no infection or pathological condition, other forms of treatment, including manipulation, may be considered. In manipulation the joint is taken to the end of its passive range of motion and then a quick thrust (high velocity and short amplitude) is applied. These techniques require a high level of skill and are applied by osteopaths and chiropractors. Physiotherapists most often use articulation in similar problems which involves moving the joint just to the end of its passive range (low velocity and high to medium amplitude). Not all of them have obtained education in this speciality as it is not included in the standard curriculum.

Many other problems and painful conditions outside the spine have vertebrogenic origins. On the other hand, many spinal problems are due to muscle imbalance and tension elsewhere in the body. Different professions have contrary opinions as to the cause and effect of such problems. Arguing this point is fruitless as it has not been possible to prove. The most effective treatment is often massage and articulation or manipulation in combination.

When conditions fail to respond fully to treatment, or if the condition recurs, this could be due to such things as poor footplant, leg length discrepancy, bad posture or poor movement patterns. It is not usually possible to correct these simply by treating secondary tension. Orthotic devices can be made by chiropodists or podiatrists to correct such things as excessive pronation, and leg length discrepancy. However, it should be pointed out that most people will have some difference in leg lengths, which cause no problems. Advice to use heel lifts should only be considered by a specialist in the subject.

Congenital or post traumatic ligament laxity can often be helped with supportive strappings which are made for different parts of the body, like ankles and knees. Their effect is two fold: they support by applying an extra tissue layer, and they also increase sensory feedback to improve coordination.

14
ACUPRESSURE THERAPY

This is a therapy which has to be studied carefully as its effects are only partly mechanical and a great deal of response is achieved through reflexes. There has been much research into the effects of acupressure, which has also helped in the understanding of similar effects with massage therapy. It would be a tremendous waste for the therapist not to use the knowledge of the complex mechanisms of the body's reflex systems which have been acquired during thousands of years of practical application. By learning to give massage in a way that stimulates these systems one can achieve better results than by just being confined to traditional Western massage, which is restricted to more mechanical effects.

'Acu' means needle and 'puncture' means sticking. Traditionally acupuncture points are stimulated in China by finger pressure, massage along the channels or by using the heat of slowly burning moxa. These are especially applied for small children and those who are afraid of needles. Massage along the channels can also be combined with needle acupuncture to reinforce the effects. It is important to note that to achieve an acupuncture effect, stimulation has to be local in whatever method is used. Generalised stimulation like pressure with a flat hand or the heat of a sauna does not produce the same effect.

Local stimulation can be applied:
• mechanically (pressure, massage and needles)
• chemically (injections)
• cold (ice)
• heat (moxa)
• electrical currents (TNS, DIDY, high voltage)
• ultrasound
• laser

TSUBO THERAPY

'Tsubos' are special sensitive spots (acupuncture points). This therapy is practically the same as acupuncture, and was developed by the Japanese who rediscovered the usefulness of the ancient Chinese therapy. There are also many other, less well known, therapies with different names which all have slightly modified approaches to the same basic principles. As every therapist develops his own style it is not surprising that so many names have evolved.

HISTORY

Acupuncture is a therapy which has been developed by one of the oldest cultures in the world. The oldest text dealing with it is a medical book by Huangdi Neijing (2697–2596 BC), *Yellow Emperor's Classic of Internal Medicine.* The book itself is estimated to have been compiled in around 500–300 BC. It still remains one of the basic references of traditional Chinese medicine, which is largely practised side by side with Western medicine in China. Acupuncture therapy today in China has changed very little and is practised in a basically similar way as it was thousands of years ago.

The Chinese have an old story about how acupuncture was discovered. It tells of a soldier who was stuck by a sword by his opponent, and due to it hitting the right point his long-standing severe disease was cured. This is a nice story, but it is more natural to assume that acupuncture developed from massage. This is because acupuncture points are easily located in the soft tissue through palpation. By treating acupuncture points one can achieve good results, not only with pain relief, but also with relaxation of muscle tension. Often when pressing 'activated' points with the finger the patient experiences a sharp pain like a needle being stuck deep through the skin. It is this which probably made the Chinese think of using needles for treatment.

Treatment methods like acupuncture have been practised in many other countries, and old maps exist showing treatment points which compare closely with those used in acupuncture. But only in China is it known to have developed as a complete healing method, and its records go back much further than any others.

TRADITIONAL THEORY

For the Chinese, the philosophy and ethics of Confucianism and the religious system of Taoism are central to their thinking. This also gives them an essential part of their traditional way of explaining the causes of diseases. For Western people who are not familiar with Chinese culture and theories of Yin and Yang and the Five Elements it all sounds rather naïve. Translations often make this worse because they make a direct comparison with Western medicine. This has led to 'cookbooks' of acupuncture, where Western diagnosis is combined with the Chinese philisophical explanation of causes and treatment of acupuncture points.

Giving treatment based on this type of approach rarely achieves good results and has done little to help the reputation of acupuncture. It has also made medical doctors sceptical about its effects, which for a long time were believed to occur merely through suggestion. For this reason acupuncture was slow to develop in Western countries until recently, when research showed that it had real effects independent of mental condition. On the contrary it has been noticed that less success is achieved when treating mentally labile and neurotic people.

EFFECTS

The most well known effect of acupuncture is its ability to abolish pain. It has been shown to release endorphins in the brain which affect the opiate receptors. This process blocks pain in a similar way to intravenously injected morphine as it is transported to the central nervous system. This explains why pain thresholds are higher throughout the whole body after acupuncture. Acupuncture also works segmentally to abolish localised pain and to create a feeling of numbness. This has been explained by 'gate control' theory: stimulation coming via thick sensory nerves from certain neurological segments inhibits pain impulses mediated by thin nerves in the posterior horns of the spinal chord. Similarly the sensation of pain is also modulated in other levels of the central nervous system.

In many cases a more important factor in diminishing pain is that acupuncture releases muscle tension. In so doing it not only relieves pain, but it also has an effect on the cause of the pain. As well as treating skeletal muscles, acupuncture is also able to affect the smooth muscles of internal organs and can give relief in conditions like gallstone and urinary stone attacks. Such effects are mediated through the autonomous nervous system. Other effects demonstrated by acupuncture are changes in: heart rate, blood pressure, peripheral circulation, intestinal motility and immunological responses.

PSAC (Propagated Sensation Along Channels)

Points and channels have been found through long practical experience. When one stimulates acupuncture points along the channels with needles, or sometimes even by pressing hard with the tip of the finger, a radiating pain may be caused. It will follow certain channels, usually stopping before the next joint, but with more sensitive people it can be felt in the whole part or through the whole channel. There can also be numbness, and hot or cold sensations experienced. This is called the PSAC phenomenon. The nerves do not run along the same routes so cannot be used to explain this phenomenon, neither can it be related to segmental innervation (with dermatomes, myotomes or sclerotomes) as their locations also differ from the channels. PSAC is a coordinated pain sensation in the central nervous system and is closely related to the somatosensory area of the cortex of the brain. It is a clearly distinct feature of the *body image*, differing from all other sensation patterns.

ACUPRESSURE TREATMENT METHOD

The pressure is applied using the thumb or finger tip moving from point to point along the part of the channel being treated. To use the elbow or knee, as in Shiatsu (see the next chapter), is too harsh, and pressure cannot be located specifically enough. With these it is more a case of inducing relaxation through general pressure. The amount of pressure applied by the finger should be moderate, and no pain sensation should be experienced when treating nor-

mal channels, although some tenderness will always exist. Pressure is increased gradually to avoid causing excessive pain, but acupressure therapy is not painless as one is often working on very sensitive spots. Channels and points which need special attention are more tender, and excessive tension is often felt in the surrounding tissues.

With traditional acupressure the direction in which one treats the channels depends on whether one aims to reinforce or decrease the Yin or Yang in that area. From clinical experience it has been found that, when treating musculoskeletal disorders, it makes no difference which direction the acupressure is applied, so channels can be stimulated in both directions. In most cases it is beneficial to start far away from a painful and tense area and gradually work towards it. This enables pain to be reduced in the affected area early in the treatment so it becomes easier as one works closer to it.

When treating abnormal conditions, pain should be kept to a bearable level. In many cases it is beneficial to leave very tender areas at peace for a while and return there after ordinary massage or after treating other channels. Often by then tenderness will have eased to some extent so one is able to give more effective treatment.

There are no strict rules about how long to apply pressure. Recommendations for the method of pressing points are often not given at all, and where they are they may vary from five seconds to one or two minutes. There is no purpose in pressing for too long as this will cause the tissues beneath to become numb through transitory ischemia. However, this can be avoided by using very local circular movements, which also acts to increase stimulation. Further benefits can be gained by massaging the channels, not just concentrating on the specific points.

The time needed for treatment will depend on the number of channels which require special attention. Time spent working on a channel will depend on a person's pain tolerance as well as the tension and tenderness along it. With local painful conditions fewer channels usually need treatment but more time can be spent on them. Channels should be treated until one can feel the tension decrease in the surrounding tissues and tenderness eases off. It is inadequate to just work quickly through a channel without responding to its condition.

Severe and long-standing conditions may require several hours of treatment to obtain really good results on the first occasion, which is often impractical. The benefits of acupressure develop over the day or two afterwards, although there will be some immediate effect. So it is better to have several treatment sessions and not try to achieve full recovery in just one long treatment. When a sportsman has little time before competition, a long session is advisable.

Acupressure therapy should be included as part of general sports massage. It should not normally take up much extra time because, when using acupressure, less effort is needed for deep massage and muscle stretching. When treating particular problems, like trauma and stiffness, the recommended frequency for treatment is twice a week. In special acute cases, treatment can be applied every day.

ACUPUNCTURE VERSUS ACUPRESSURE

When comparing these two therapies one cannot simply say which is more effective. Much depends on how the therapy is performed as well as on each individual case. With acupuncture one achieves a stronger stimulation in certain local points as the needle penetrates deeply into the tissue and causes microtrauma. There are cases where acupuncture is better than massage, such as in pain due to tension in deep back and buttock muscles.

Acupressure has its own advantages by working through whole channels rather than selected points along them. Massage also has the advantage that one is constantly looking for tender areas and points (Ahshi points), which may otherwise go unnoticed by the acupuncturist who only uses needles.

For this reason acupressure restricted only to the channels, or even worse to just some points, should not be used as the only treatment. It is complementary to massage and cannot replace it. To do so would be to miss out on the diagnostic and mechanical benefits of massage.

LOCALISATION OF THE ACUPUNCTURE POINTS

Anatomical landmarks

Feeling muscles, tendons and bones while massaging is the most accurate way to locate channels and acupuncture points. Channels are easy to locate because they are often on the border of the muscles and bones. Acupuncture points are not always close to easily felt prominent structures, but they are often found by their distinct sensitivity to pressure from the fingers moving along the channel, especially in problem areas.

Finger measurement

This method is used most commonly when locating points on the channel where there are no proper anatomical landmarks. The unit of measurement is dependent on the hand size of the person being treated, and, if this differs much from the size of the therapist's hand, this should be taken into account.

1 cun is the breadth of the interphalangeal joint of the thumb

2 cun is the breadth of the distal interphalangal joints, when the fingers are slightly apart

3 cun is the breadth of hand at the level of proximal interphalangeal joints (midway)

Proportional measurement

The diagram on p. 122 shows some proportional measures. These distances are then divided into units to locate the points. One can use a rubber band which is marked at regular intervals (1 cun), which can then be stretched according to the size of the person being treated by first taking a measurement from a known distance. However, finger measurement is the quickest when one has become accustomed to using it. It is also more accurate as one can take anatomical landmarks nearby as a measuring point.

Electrical devices

Studies have shown that electrical resistance of the skin is lower at acupuncture points than in the surrounding skin. There are several electronic devices on the market which are meant to locate and treat the points using this method. Most of these are, however, of no value, and they can be very expensive. Even if one could get proper instruments for this purpose, it would take too long for the therapist to locate the points. This is because the skin's electrical resistance varies in different areas, and the device would need to be tuned specifically for each area. The therapist has to learn where points and channels are located if one wants to use acupressure as a part of massage.

ACUPRESSURE POINTS

In the following are listed the points of twelve regular channels and two extra channels. There are four more extra channels, but these do not have their own points (they run along part of the regular channels). The location of channel points are listed below. For sports therapists using massage it is not necessary to memorise the exact locations of the points. One should go through the points in order to learn the location of channels. In musculoskeletal disorders the channels of most importance are the large intestine channel for the arms, and spleen, stomach, gall bladder and urinary bladder channels for the legs. Points will be easily found when treating the channels. If the channels cannot be localised automatically from memory, it is not possible to use acupressure therapy effectively.

The lung channel (Lu)

Lu 1. Between the 1st and 2nd ribs, 6 cun lateral to the midline.

Lu 2. Between clavicle and 1st rib, 6 cun lateral to the midline.

Lu 3. Between the two parts of biceps muscle, 3 cun below the armpit fold.

Lu 4. Between the two parts of biceps muscle, 4 cun below the armpit fold.

Lu 5. In the cubital crease, on the radial side of tendon of biceps muscle.

Lu 6. 7 cun above the crease of the wrist, between the brachioradialis and pronator teres muscles.

Lu 7. Just above the styloid process of the radius.

Lu 8. 1 cun above transverse crease of the wrist, in the palmar side of the styloid process of the radius.

Lu 9. In transverse crease of the wrist, on the radial side of the radial artery.

Lu 10. In the middle of the first metacarpal bone on the border of palmar and dorsal skin.

Lu 11. 0.1 cun from the radial corner of the nail of the thumb.

Acupressure measurement unit

'Cun' is a proportional measurement unit, depending on
the size of the person being treated.

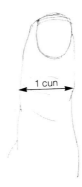

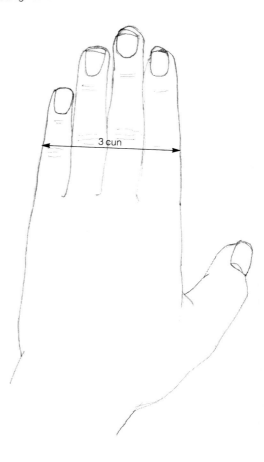

* 1 cun is the breadth of the thumb at the level of the
interphalangeal joint.

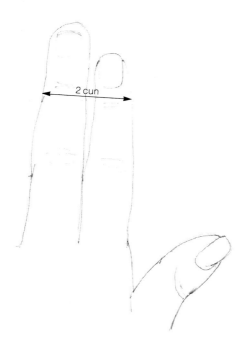

***3 cun is the breadth from the 2nd to the 5th fingers
at the level of the proximal interphalangeal joint.

** 2 cun is the breadth of the index and forefinger at the
level of the interphalangeal joint, when the fingers are
slightly apart.

15　Acupressure measurement chart

The pericardium channel (P)

P. 1. In the 4th intercostal space, 1 cun lateral to the nipple.

P. 2. Between the biceps brachii and coraco-brachialis muscles, 2 cun below the axillary fold.

P. 3. In the transverse cubital crease, at the ulnar side of biceps brachii tendon.

P. 4. 5 cun above the transverse crease of the wrist, between the tendons of the palmaris longus and flexor carpi radialis.

P. 5. 3 cun above the transverse crease of the wrist, between the tendons of the palmaris longus and flexor carpi radialis.

P. 6. 2 cun above the crease of the wrist, between the tendons of the palmaris longus and flexor carpi radialis.

P. 7. At transverse crease of the wrist, between the tendons of the palmaris longus and flexor carpi radialis.

P. 8. Over the 3rd metacarpal bone, in the upper transverse crease of the palm.

P. 9. At the midpoint of the tip of the middle finger.

The heart channel (H)

H. 1. At the centre of the axillary fossa, on the front of the axillary artery.

H. 2. 3 cun above crease of the elbow joint, between the biceps brachii and brachialis muscles.

H. 3. Halfway between the medial end of the transverse cubital crease and the medial epicondyle of the humerus, when the elbow joint is fully bent.

H. 4. 1.5 cun above the palmar fold of the wrist, on the radial side of the flexor carpi ulnaris tendon.

H. 5. 1 cun above the palmar fold of the wrist, on the radial side of the flexor carpi ulnaris tendon.

H. 6. 0.5 cun above the palmar fold of the wrist, on the radial side of the flexor carpi ulnaris tendon.

H. 7. In the palmar fold of the wrist, on the radial side of the flexor carpi ulnaris tendon.

H. 8. The palmar surface of the hand between and midway along the 4th and 5th meta-carpal bones, on the upper transverse line.

H. 9. 0.1 cun posterior to the radial corner of the nail of the small finger.

The large intestine channel (L.I.)

L.I. 1 0.1 cun from the radial corner of the nail of the index finger.

L.I. 2. In the depression distal metacarpo-phalangeal joint of the index finger on the radial side, in the junction of palmar and dorsal skin.

L.I. 3. The depression proximal to the meta-carpophalangeal joint of index finger, in the junction of palmar and dorsal skin.

L.I. 4. Halfway between the 1st and 2nd meta-carpal bones of the index finger.

L.I. 5. Midway between the tendons of the extensor pollicus brevis and longus muscles, on the wrist joint.

L.I. 6. 3 cun above the wrist joint, on the ulnar side of the tendon of the extensor carpi radialis brevis muscle.

L.I. 7. 5 cun above the wrist joint, on the ulnar side of extensor carpi radialis brevis muscle.

L.I. 8. 4 cun below the elbow crease, on the ulnar side of the extensor carpi radialis longus muscle.

L.I. 9. 3 cun below the cubital crease, on the ulnar side of extensor carpi radialis longus muscle.

L.I. 10. 2 cun below the cubital crease, on the ulnar side of extensor carpi radialis longus muscle.

L.I. 11. In the lateral end of the transverse cubital crease when the elbow is flexed to a right angle.

L.I. 12. 1 cun above the cubital crease, on the lateral border of triceps muscle.

L.I. 13. 3 cun above the elbow crease, on the lateral border of brachialis muscle.

L.I. 14. On the attachment of deltoid muscle in the midway along the humerus.

L.I. 15. Below the acromion, between the front and middle part of the deltoid muscle.

L.I. 16. In the depression behind the acromio-clavicular joint.

L.I. 17. 1 cun below L.I. 18, at the posterior border of sternocleidomastoid muscle.

L.I. 18. Midway between two ends of sterno-cleidomastoid muscle, on a level with the prominence of the thyroid cartilage (Adam's apple), in the middle of the muscle.

L.I. 19. In the middle of upper lip, straight below the lateral ala of the nose.

L.I. 20. In the nasolabial groove on a level with the opening of the nostril.

The sanjiao channel (S.J.)

S.J. 1. 0.1 cun proximal to the ulnar corner of the nail of the 4th finger.

S.J. 2. In the depression distal to the 4th metacarpophalangeal joint, on the ulnar side.

S.J. 3. In the depression proximal to the 4th metacarpophalangeal joint, on the ulnar side.

S.J. 4. In the depression between the tendons of the extensor digitorum communis and extensor digiti minimi, in the transverse crease of the wrist.

S.J. 5. 2 cun above the transverse crease of the wrist, between the radius and ulna.

S.J. 6. 3 cun above transverse crease of the wrist, between the radius and ulnar.

S.J. 7. 3 cun above the transverse crease of the wrist, one finger breadth lateral to S.J. 6.

S.J. 8. 4 cun above the transverse crease of the wrist, between the radius and ulna.

S.J. 9. 5 cun below the proximal border of the olecranon process, between the radius and ulna.

S.J. 10. 1 cun above the olecranon process, in the depression in the middle on the tendon of the triceps muscle felt when the elbow joint is flexed.

S.J. 11. 2 cun above the olecranon process, in the depression in the middle on the tendon of triceps muscle felt when elbow joint is flexed.

S.J. 12. 6 cun below acromion, on the posterior border of the lateral head of the triceps brachii muscle.

S.J. 13. 3 cun below acromion, on the posterior border of the deltoid muscle.

S.J. 14. In the depression between posterior and middle part of deltoid muscle, below the acromion.

S.J. 15. Midway between interspinous space C7-Th1 and the tip of the acromion. In the depression in the trapezius muscle 1 cun posterior to G.B. 21.

S.J. 16. On the posterior border of the sternocleidomastoid muscle, in the level of the lower border of the mandible.

S.J. 17. In the depression between the mandible bone and mastoid process, beneath the ear lobe.

S.J. 18. Posterior to the ear lobe, 1 cun above S.J. 17.

S.J. 19. Posterior to the ear lobe, 2 cun above S.J. 17.

S.J. 20. Just inside the hairline, level with the tip of the ear lobe.

S.J. 21. In the depression in front of the anterior notch of the auricle, 0.5 finger breadth above zygomatic bone.

S.J. 22. On the posterior hairline, slightly above S.J. 21.

S.J. 23. In the notch on the lateral border of the orbit at the tip of the eyebrow.

The small intestine channel (S.I.)

S.I. 1. 0.1 cun posterior to the ulnar corner of the nail of the small finger.

S.I. 2. In the depression distal to the 5th metacarpophalangal joint in the junction of palmar and dorsal skin.

S.I. 3. In the depression proximal to the 5th metacarpophalangeal joint in the junction of the palmar and dorsal skin.

S.I. 4. In the depression between the 5th metacarpal bone and the hamate bone in the junction of palmar and dorsal skin.

S.I. 5. In the depression between the styloid process and pisiform bone in the junction of palmar and dorsal skin.

S.I. 6. In the depression proximal to the radial side of the head of the ulna.

S.I. 7. 5 cun proximal to the wrist joint, in the border of the ulna.

S.I. 8. In the groove under the medial epicondyle.

S.I. 9. 1 cun superior to the posterior axillary fold.

S.I. 10. Directly above the posterior axillary fold, on the lower border of the spine of the scapula.

S.I. 11. In the centre of the infrascapular fossa and the highest point of infraspinatus muscle.

S.I. 12. In the notch on the upper border of scapula.

S.I. 13. In medial end of the subscapular fossa, midway between S.I. 10 and the 2nd thoracic vertebra.

S.I. 14. In upper medial corner of scapula on the attachment of levator scapulae muscle.

S.I. 15. 2 cun lateral to the lower border of the 7th cervical spinous process.

S.I. 16. On the posterior border of the sternocleidomastoid muscle, midway between the attachments, on a level with the prominence of the thyroid cartilage (Adam's apple).

S.I. 17. On the anterior border of the sternocleidomastoid, on the level of lower border of the jaw.

S.I. 18. In the depression anteriorily on lower margin of the zygomatic bone, below outer canthus of eye.

S.I. 19. In the depression between the tragus and mandibular joint, which appears as mouth is opened.

The spleen channel (Sp)

Sp. 1. 0.1 cun posterior to the medial corner of the nail of the big toe.

Sp. 2. In the depression distal to the 1st metatarsophalangeal joint, in the junction of plantar and dorsal skin.

Sp. 3. In the depression proximal to the 1st metatarsophalangeal joint, in the junction of plantar and dorsal skin.

Sp. 4. In the depression distal to the joint between the metatarsal and medial cuneiform bones, in the junction of the plantar and dorsal skin.

Sp. 5. In the depression of the ankle joint, on the medial side of the tibialis anterior tendon.

Sp. 6. 3 cun above the tip of the medial malleolus, just posterior to the tibial border.

Sp. 7. 6 cun above the tip of the medial malleolus, just posterior to the border of the tibia.

Sp. 8. 6 cun below the lower border of the patella, at the posterior border of the tibia.

Sp. 9. In the depression below the medial condyle, at the posterior border of the tibia.

Sp. 10. 2 cun above the superior border of the patella, in the middle of vastus medialis muscle.

Sp. 11. 8 cun above the superior border of the patella, on the medial border of the sartorius muscle.

Sp. 12. In the fold of the groin, on the lateral side of the femoral artery.

Sp. 13. 1 cun above the upper border of the symphysis pubis, 4 cun lateral to the midline (in the lateral border of rectus abdominis muscle).

Sp. 14. 1.3 cun below the navel, 4 cun lateral to the midline.

Sp. 15. 4 cun lateral to the umbilicus.

Sp. 16. 3 cun above the navel, 4 cun lateral to the midline.

Sp. 17. 5th intercostal space, 6 cun from midline.

Sp. 18. 4th intercostal space, 6 cun from midline (2 cun lateral to mamilla).

Sp. 19. 3rd intercostal space, 6 cun from midline.

Sp. 20. 2nd intercostal space, 6 cun from midline.

Sp. 21. 6th intercostal space, on the midaxillary line.

The liver channel (Liv.)

Liv. 1. 0.1 cun posterior to the lateral corner of the nail of the 1st toe.

Liv. 2. In the cleft distal to the 1st metatarsophalangeal joint.

Liv. 3. In the cleft proximal to the 1st metatarsophalangeal joint on the lateral side.

Liv. 4. In the depression of the ankle joint, between the extensor tibialis anterior and hallucis longus tendons.

Liv. 5. On the posterior border of the tibia, 5 cun above the tip of the medial malleolus.

Liv. 6. On the posterior border of the tibia, 7 cun above the tip of the medial malleolus.

Liv. 7. 1 cun from the depression below the medial epicondyle (Sp. 9) in a superior and posterior direction of its border.

Liv. 8. In the depression between the gracilis and semimembrinosus tendons at the level with the transverse crease of the knee.

Liv. 9. 4 cun above the upper border of the patella, in the depression between the quadriceps and sartorius muscles.

Liv. 10. Between the femoral artery and sartorius muscle, 2 cun below the inguinal groove.

Liv. 11. On the lateral side of the femoral artery, 1 cun below inguinal groove.

Liv. 12. 1 cun below and 2.5 cun lateral to the superior border of the pubic symphysis, in the inguinal groove.

Liv. 13. At the free end of the 11th rib.

Liv. 14. In the 6th intercostal space, on the mammillary line.

The kidney channel (K)

K. 1. In the depression between the 2nd and 3rd metatarsal bones at the junction of the distal and middle third of the sole.

K. 2. In the depression at the joint between the medial cuneiform and navicular bone, in the junction of the plantar and dorsal skin.

K. 3. Midway between the calcaneus tendon and the tip of the medial malleolus.

K. 4. In the depression in front of the calcaneus tendon attachment, 1 cun below and 0.5 cun posterior to K. 3.

K. 5. 1 cun directly inferior to K. 3.

K. 6. In the depression 1 cun below the inferior border of the medial malleolus.

K. 7. 2 cun above the tip of the medial malleolus on the anterior border of the calcaneus tendon.

K. 8. In the depression posterior to the medial tibial border, 2 cun above the tip of the medial malleolus.

K. 9. 1 cun posterior to the medial tibial border, 5 cun above the tip of the medial malleolus.

K. 10. Between the semimembranosus and semitendinosus tendons, at the level of the popliteal transverse crease.

K. 11. On the superior border of the pubic symphysis, 0.5 cun from the midline.

K. 12. 1 cun above the pubic symphysis, 0.5 cun lateral to midline.

K. 13. 2 cun above the pubic symphysis, 0.5 cun lateral to midline.

K. 14. 2 cun below the umbilicus, 0.5 cun lateral to midline.

K. 15. 1 cun below the umbilicus, 0.5 cun lateral to midline.

K. 16. 0.5 cun lateral to the umbilicus.

K. 17. 2 cun above the umbilicus, 0.5 cun lateral to midline.

K. 18. 3 cun above the umbilicus, 0.5 cun lateral to midline.

K.19. 4 cun above the umbilicus, 0.5 cun lateral to midline.

K. 20. 5 cun above the umbilicus, 0.5 cun lateral to midline.

K. 21. 6 cun above the umbilicus, 0.5 cun lateral to midline.

K. 22. In the 5th intercostal space, 2 cun from midline.

K. 23. In the 4th intercostal space, 2 cun from midline.

K. 24. In the 3rd intercostal space, 2 cun from midline.

K. 25. In the 2nd intercostal space, 2 cun from midline.

K. 26. In the 1st intercostal space, 2 cun from midline.

K. 27. In the depression between the clavicle and the 1st rib, 2 cun from the midline.

The stomach channel (St)

St. 1. In the middle of upper border of the infra-orbital ridge.

St. 2. A finger's breadth below St. 1, at the depression of the infra-orbital foramen.

St. 3. Below St. 2, on the lower border of the maxillary bone.

St. 4. 0.5 cun lateral to the corner of the mouth.

St. 5. In the lower border of jaw, on the front border of masseter muscle.

St. 6. One finger breadth anterior from the back border of mandible bone and one finger breadth above the lower border of mandible.

St. 7. In the depression at the lower border of the zygomatic arch, in front of the mandible condyle.

St. 8. At the corner of the forehead, where the frontal, temporal and parietal bones join, 3.5 cun above the eyebrow.

St. 9. On the anterior border of the sternocleido-mastoid, posterior to the common carotid artery at the level of the most prominent area of thyroid cartilage (Adam's apple).

St. 10. Anterior border of the sternocleido-mastoid midway between St. 9 and St. 11.

St. 11. Superior border of the clavicle directly below St. 9.

St. 12. Superior border of the clavicle, on the mammary line.

St. 13. Inferior border of the clavicle, on the mammary line.

St. 14. 1st intercostal space, on the mammary line (4 cun lateral to midline).

St. 15. 2nd intercostal space, on the mammary line.

St. 16. 3rd intercostal space, on the mammary line.

St. 17. 4th intercostal space, in the mammary nipple.

St. 18. 5th intercostal space, in the mammary line.

St. 19. 6 cun above the umbilicus, 2 cun from midline.

St. 20. 5 cun above the umbilicus, 2 cun from midline.

St. 21. 4 cun above the umbilicus, 2 cun from midline.

St. 22. 3 cun above the umbilicus, 2 cun from midline.

St. 23. 2 cun above umbilicus, 2 cun from midline.

St. 24. 1 cun above umbilicus, 2 cun from midline.

St. 25. On the level of the umbilicus, 2 cun from midline.

St. 26. 1 cun below umbilicus, 2 cun from midline.

St. 27. 2 cun below umbilicus, 2 cun from midline.

St. 28. 2 cun above pubic bone, 2 cun from midline.

St. 29. 1 cun above pubic bone, 2 cun from midline.

St. 30. Upper border of pubic bone, 2 cun from midline.

St. 31. Directly below the superior anterior iliac spine, between the rectus femoris and tensor fascia lata muscles, on the level of the lower border of symphysis pubis.

St. 32. 6 cun above the superior border of the patella, on the lateral border of the rectus femoris muscle.

St. 33. 3 cun above the superior lateral border of the patella, on the lateral border of rectus femoris muscle.

St. 34. 2 cun above the superior lateral border of the patella, on the lateral border of rectus femoris muscle.

St. 35. In the depression just below the patella, lateral to the patella ligament.

St. 36. 3 cun below the lower border of the patella, one finger breadth lateral to the anterior crest of tibia, in the middle of the tibialis anterior muscle.

St. 37. 6 cun below the lower border of the patella, one finger breadth lateral to the anterior crest of tibia.

St. 38. 8 cun below the lower border of the patella, one finger breadth lateral to the anterior crest of tibia.

St. 39. 9 cun below the lower border of the patella, one finger breadth lateral to the anterior crest of tibia.

St. 40. 8 cun below the lower border of the patella, two finger breadths lateral to the anterior crest of tibia, on the lateral border of the tibialis anterior muscle.

St. 41. At transverse crease of ankle joint, between the extensor digitorum longus and hallicus longus tendons.

St. 42. In the depression between medial cuneiform, and 1st and 2nd metatarsal bones.

St. 43. In the depression proximal to the 1st metatarsophalangeal joint on the lateral side.

St. 44. In the depression distal to the 2nd metatarsophalangeal joint on the lateral side.

St. 45. 0.1 cun proximal to the lateral corner of the nail of the second toe.

The gall bladder channel (G.B.)

G.B. 1. On the border of the orbit, 0.5 cun lateral to the canthus.

G.B. 2. In front of the ear lobe, at level of the lower border of tragus.

G.B. 3. In front of the ear lobe, on the upper border of the zygomatic arch, directly above St. 7.

G.B. 4. 1 cun below the prominence on forehead, where frontal, parietal and temporal bones join (St. 8), 2.5. cun above the eyebrow.

G.B. 5. Between the upper and middle third from G.B. 4 to G.B. 7.

G.B. 6. Between the middle and lower third from G.B. 4 to G.B. 7.

G.B. 7. At the point where the horizontal line of the upper border and the vertical line of the front border of auricular lobe meet.

G.B. 8. Directly above the apex of the auricle, 1.5. cun inside the hairline.

G.B. 9. 0.5 cun posterior to G.B. 8, 2 cun inside the hairline.

G.B. 10. 1 cun below G.B. 9, at the upper border of the root of the auricle, 1 cun inside the hairline.

G.B. 11. Midway between G.B. 10 and G.B. 12.

G.B. 12. In the depression back and below the mastoid process.

G.B. 13. Directly above the outer canthus, 3.5 cun above the eyebrow.

G.B. 14. 1 cun above the midpoint of the eyebrow.

G.B. 15. Above G.B. 14, 3.5 cun within the hairline.

G.B. 16. 1 cun posterior to G.B. 15.

G.B. 17. 1 cun posterior to G.B. 16.

G.B. 18. 1 cun posterior to G.B. 17.

G.B. 19. 1 cun above G.B. 20, on the lateral side of the occipital protuberance.

G.B. 20. In the depression below the occipital bone between the sternocleidomastoid and trapezius muscle.

G.B. 21. Midway between the interspinous space C7-Th1 and the tip of acromion, at the highest point of the shoulder.

G.B. 22. On the axillary line, in the 4th intercostal space.

G.B. 23. 1 cun anterior to G.B. 22 in the 4th intercostal space.

G.B. 24. In the 7th intercostal space, on the mamillary line.

G.B. 25. At the lower border of the tip of the 12th rib.

G.B. 26. Level with the umbilicus, midway between the tips of the 11th and 12th ribs.

G.B. 27. In front of the superior inferior iliac spine, 2 cun above the symphysis pubis.

G.B. 28. 0.5 cun downwards and forwards from G.B. 27, in front of the superior iliac spine.

G.B. 29. In the posterior border of tensor faciae latae muscle, midway between the top of the great trochanter of the femur and the anterior superior iliac spine.

G.B. 30. At the junction of middle and lateral third from the top of the great trochanter to the hiatus of the sacrum.

G.B. 31. 7 cun above the transverse popliteal crease, between the quadriceps and biceps femoris muscles.

G.B. 32. 5 cun above the transverse popliteal crease, between the quadriceps and biceps femoris muscles.

G.B. 33. In the depression above the lateral epicondyle of the femur, between the quadriceps muscle and biceps femoris tendon.

G.B. 34. In the depression below the head of the fibula on the front side.

G.B. 35. 7 cun above the tip of the lateral malleolus, on the anterior border of the fibula.

G.B. 36. 7 cun above the tip of the lateral malleolus, on the posterior border of the fibula.

G.B. 37. 5 cun above the tip of the lateral malleolus, on the anterior border of the fibula.

G.B. 38. 4 cun above the tip of the lateral malleolus, on the anterior border of the fibula.

G.B. 39. 3 cun above the tip of the lateral malleolus, on the posterior border of the fibula.

G.B. 40. In the depression of the ankle joint, behind the extensor digitorum longus tendon.

G.B. 41. In the depression anterior to the junction of the 4th and 5th metatarsal bones.

G.B. 42. In the cleft on the lateral side proximal to the 4th metatarsophalangeal joint.

G.B. 43. In the cleft on the lateral side distal to the 4th metatarsophalangeal joint.

G.B. 44. 0.1 cun posterior to the lateral corner of the nail of the 4th toe.

The urinary bladder channel of the foot (U.B.)

U.B. 1. Above the inner canthus of the eye.

U.B. 2. On the supraorbital margin in the depression at the medial end of the eyebrow.

U.B. 3. 3.5. cun above the eyebrow, 0.5. cun lateral to the midline.

U.B. 4. 3.5 cun above the eyebrow, 1.5. cun lateral to the midline.

U.B. 5. 0.5 cun posterior to U.B. 4.

U.B. 6. 1.5 cun posterior to U.B. 5.

U.B. 7. 1.5 cun posterior to U.B. 6.

U.B. 8. 1.5 cun posterior to U.B. 7.

U.B. 9. On the upper border of the occipital protuberance, 1.3 cun lateral to the midline.

U.B. 10. Under the occipital base, on the lateral side of the trapezius muscle tendon.

U.B. 11. In the level of interspinal space Th1-2, 1.5 cun from midline.

U.B. 12. In the level of interspinal space Th2-3, 1.5 cun from midline.

U.B. 13. In the level of interspinal space Th3-4, 1.5 cun from midline.

U.B. 14. In the level of interspinal space Th4-5, 1.5 cun from midline.

U.B. 15. In the level of interspinal space Th5-6, 1.5 cun from midline.

U.B. 16. In the level of interspinal space Th6-7, 1.5 cun from midline.

U.B. 17. In the level of interspinal space Th7-8, 1.5 cun from midline.

U.B. 18. In the level of interspinal space Th9-10, 1.5 cun from midline.

U.B. 19. In the level of interspinal space Th10-11, 1.5 cun from midline.

U.B. 20. In the level of interspinal space Th11-12, 1.5 cun from midline.

U.B. 21. In the level of interspinal space Th12-L1, 1.5 cun from midline.

U.B. 22. In the level of interspinal space L1-2, 1.5 cun from midline.

U.B. 23. In the level of interspinal space L2-3, 1.5 cun from midline.

U.B. 24. In the level of interspinal space L3-4, 1.5 cun from midline.

U.B. 25. In the level of interspinal space L4-5, 1.5 cun from midline.

U.B. 26. In the level of interspinal space L5-S1, 1.5 cun from midline.

U.B. 27. In the level of 1st sacral foramen, 1.5 cun from midline.

U.B. 28. In the level of 2nd sacral foramen, 1.5 cun from midline.

U.B. 29. In the level of 3rd sacral foramen, 1.5 cun from midline.

U.B. 30. In the level of 4th sacral foramen, 1.5 cun from midline.

U.B. 31. In the depression of the 1st sacral foramen, midway from the midline to the posterior superior iliac spine.

U.B. 32. In the depression of 2nd posterior sacral foramen.

U.B. 33. In the depression of 3rd posterior sacral foramen.

U.B. 34. In the depression of 4th posterior sacral foramen.

U.B. 35. In the lower end of the coccyx, 0.5 cun lateral to the midline.

U.B. 36. In the gluteal fold, in the middle of thigh, lateral to biceps femoris muscle.

U.B. 37. 6 cun below the gluteal fold, between the semitendinosus and biceps femoris muscles.

U.B. 38. 1 cun above the transverse popliteal crease, on the medial side of biceps femoris tendon.

U.B. 39. In the transverse popliteal crease, on the medial side of the biceps femoris tendon.

U.B. 40. In the middle of the transverse popliteal crease.

U.B. 41. In the level of interspinal space Th2-3, 3 cun from midline.

U.B. 42. In the level of interspinal space Th3-4, 3 cun from midline.

U.B. 43. In the level of interspinal space Th4-5, 3 cun from midline.

U.B. 44. In the level of interspinal space Th5-6, 3 cun from midline.

U.B. 45. In the level of interspinal space Th6-7, 3 cun from midline.

U.B. 46. In the level of interspinal space Th7-8, 3 cun from midline.

U.B. 47. In the level of interspinal space Th9-10, 3 cun from midline.

U.B. 48. In the level of interspinal space Th10-11, 3 cun from midline.

U.B. 49. In the level of interspinal space Th11-12, 3 cun from midline.

U.B. 50. In the level of interspinal space Th12-L1, 3 cun from midline.

U.B. 51. In the level of interspinal space L1-2, 3 cun from midline.

U.B. 52. In the level of interspinal space L2-3, 3 cun from midline.

U.B. 53. In the level with 2nd sacral foramen, 3 cun from midline.

U.B. 54. In the level with 4th sacral foramen, 3 cun from midline.

U.B. 55. 2 cun below the transverse popliteal crease, between the two parts of the gastrocnemius muscle.

U.B. 56. 5 cun below the transverse popliteal crease, between the two parts of gastrocnemius muscle.

U.B. 57. 8 cun below the transverse popliteal crease, between the two parts of the gastrocnemius muscle.

U.B. 58. 7 cun above the tip of lateral malleous, between the peroneus longus and soleus muscles.

U.B. 59. 3 cun above the tip of the lateral malleolus, between the peroneus longus and soleus muscles.

U.B. 60. Between the tip of the lateral malleolus and the calcaneus tendon.

U.B. 61. 1.5 cun directly below U.B. 60, at the junction of the plantar and dorsal skin.

U.B. 62. 0.5 cun directly below the lower border of the lateral malleolus.

U.B. 63. In the depression proximal to the joint between calcaneum and cuboid bones, at the junction of plantar and dorsal skin.

U.B. 64. In the depression distal to the joint between cuboid and 5th metatarsal bones, at the junction of the plantar and dorsal skin.

U.B. 65. In the depression proximal to metatarsophalangeal joint, at the junction of the plantar and dorsal skin.

U.B. 66. In the depression distal to the metatarsophalangeal joint at the junction of dorsal and plantar skin.

U.B. 67. 0.1 cun proximal to the lateral corner of the nail of the 5th toe.

The renmai channel (Ren)

Ren 1. In the centre of the perineum.

Ren 2. At the superior border of the pubic symphysis.

Ren 3. 1 cun above the border of the pubic symphysis.

Ren 4. 2 cun above the border of the pubic symphysis.

Ren 5. 2 cun below the umbilicus.

Ren 6. 1.5 cun below the umbilicus.

Ren 7. 1 cun below the umbilicus.

Ren 8. In the centre of the umbilicus.

Ren 9. 1 cun above the umbilicus.

Ren 10. 2 cun above the umbilicus.

Ren 11. 3 cun above the umbilicus.

Ren 12. 4 cun above the umbilicus.

Ren 13. 3 cun below the body of manubrium sterni.

Ren 14. 2 cun below the body of manubrium sterni.

Ren 15. 1 cun below the body of manubrium sterni.

Ren 16. In the midline, at the level of the 5th intercostal space.

Ren 17. Midway between the nipples, at a level of the 4th intercostal space.

Ren 18. In the midline, at the level of the 3rd intercostal space.

Ren 19. In the midline, at the level of the 2nd intercostal space.

Ren 20. In the midline, at the junction of the manubrium and the body of sternum.

Ren 21. In the midline, 1 cun below upper border of the sternum.

Ren 22. In the midline, on the upper border of the sternum.

Ren 23. In the midline on the upper border of hyoid bone.

Ren 24. In the middle in the mental labial groove.

The back midline channel (Du.)

Du. 1. Midway between the anus and coccyx.

Du. 2. In the hiatus of the sacrum.

Du. 3. In the interspinal space of L4-5.

Du. 4. In the interspinal space of L2-3.

Du. 5. In the interspinal space of L1-2.

Du. 6. In the interspinal space of Th11-12.

Du. 7. In the interspinal space of Th10-11.

Du. 8. In the interspinal space of Th9-10.

Du. 9. In the interspinal space of Th7-8.

Du. 10. In the interspinal space of Th6-7.

Du. 11. In the interspinal space of Th5-6.

Du. 12. In the interspinal space of Th3-4.

Du. 13. In the interspinal space of Th1-2.

Du. 14. In the interspinal space of C7-Th1.

Du. 15. In the interspinal space of C1-2.

Du. 16. Directly below the occipital bone in the midline.

Du. 17. Above the occipital protuberance, 1.5 cun above Du. 16, in the midline.

Du. 18. 3 cun above Du. 16, and below Du. 20, in the midline.

Du. 19. 1.5 cun below Du. 20, in the midline.

Du. 20. In the prominence where the occipital and parietal bones join.

Du. 21. 1.5 cun anterior to Du. 20, in the midline.

Du. 22. 3 cun anterior to Du. 20, in the midline.

Du. 23. 4 cun anterior to Du. 20, in the midline.

Du. 24. 3.5 cun above the eyebrow in the midline.

Du. 25. At the tip of the nose.

Du. 26. At the junction of upper and lower two thirds of the upper lip, in the midline.

Du. 27. On the median tubercle of the upper lip.

Du. 28. In the upper labial frenum.

Acupressure points

P   1
K   11-27
Liv   12-14
Ren   22-24
Du   24-27

Acupressure points

Lu   1-2
Sp   12-21
St   1-30
Ren 2-21

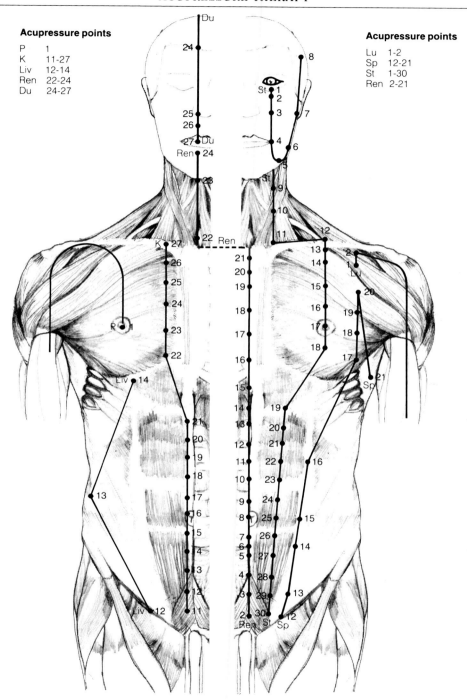

16   Acupressure chart 1

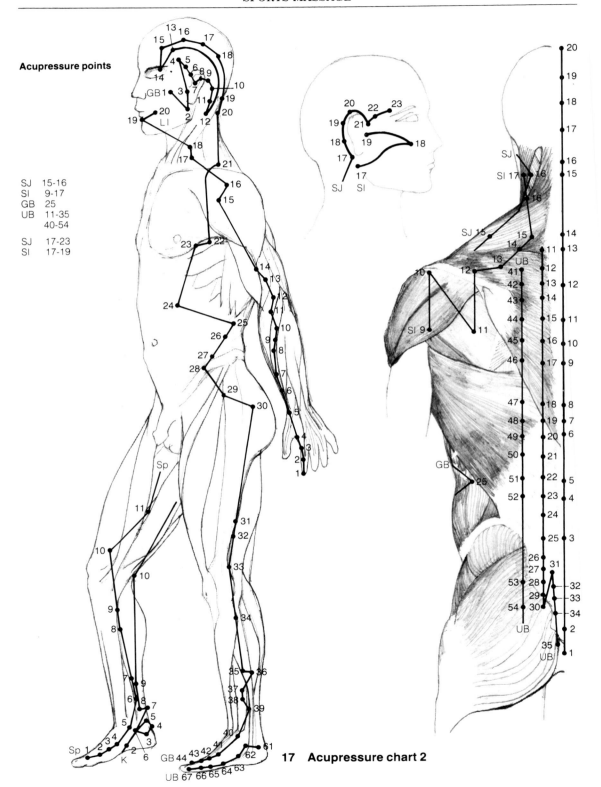

Acupressure points

SJ 15-16
SI 9-17
GB 25
UB 11-35
40-54

SJ 17-23
SI 17-19

17 Acupressure chart 2

Acupressure points

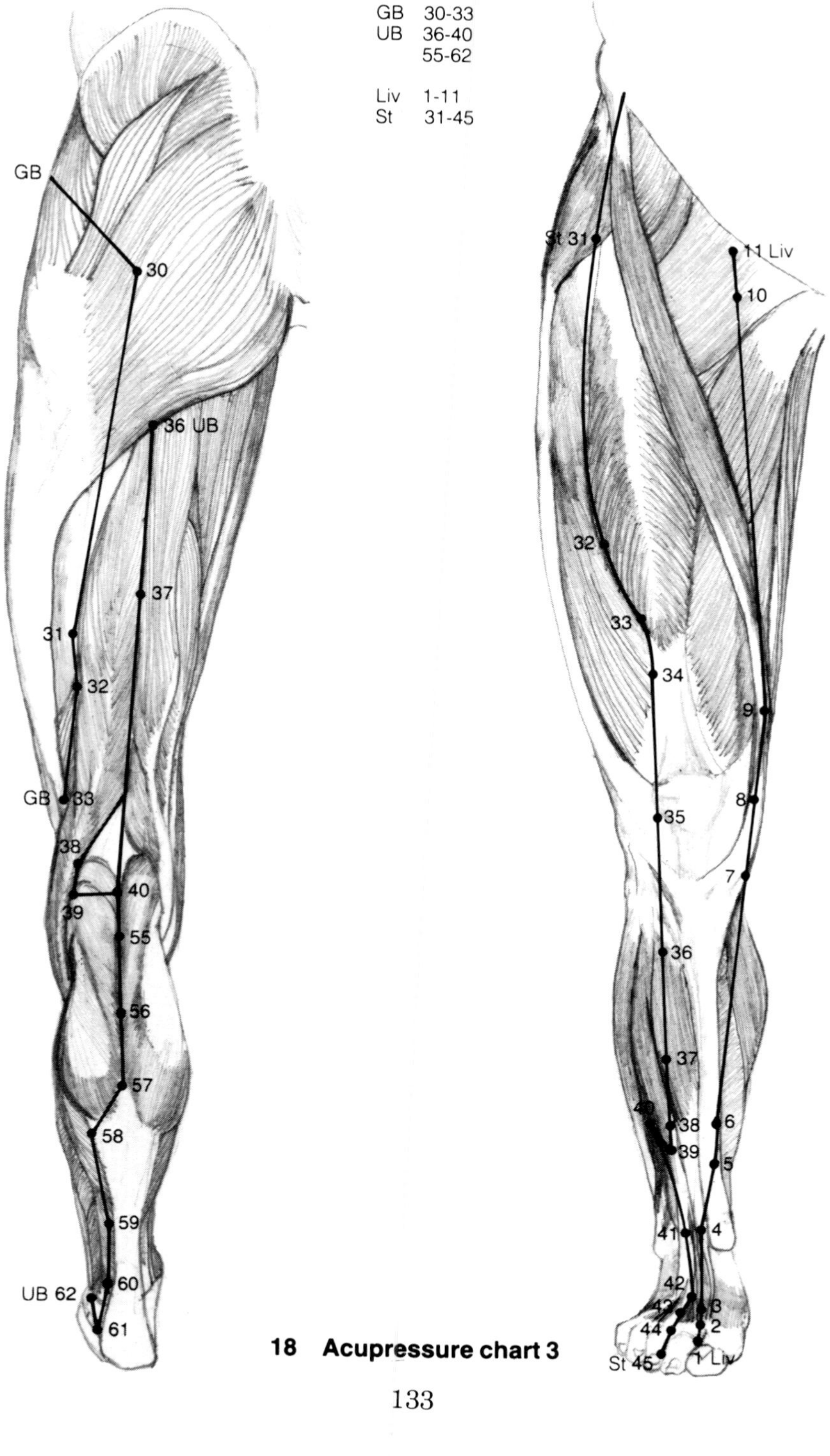

GB	30-33
UB	36-40
	55-62
Liv	1-11
St	31-45

GB

30

36 UB

37

31

32

GB 33

38

39 40

55

56

57

58

59

60

UB 62

61

St 31

11 Liv

10

32

33

34

9

8

35

7

36

37

4 38 6

39 5

41 4

42

43 3

2

44

St 45 1 Liv

18   Acupressure chart 3

133

Acupressure points

Lu	3-11
P	2-9
H	1-9
LI	1-7
SJ	1-14
SI	1-10

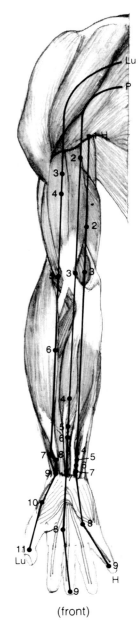

(front)

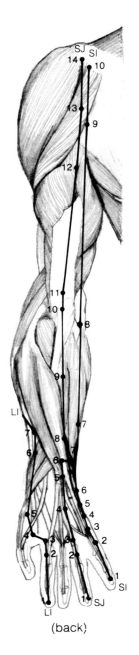

(back)

19 Acupressure chart 4

134

15
SHIATSU

This is a Japanese form of therapy which has developed in the twentieth century. 'Shi' means fingers and 'atsu' means pressure. It originates partly from ancient Eastern massage and manipulation techniques (Anma) and partly from Western massage and stretching methods. After rediscovering acupressure therapy the Japanese soon understood the value of it and developed Shiatsu therapy, which quickly became popular. It later spread to many other countries, especially the USA, where massage has not received the same status as traditional treatment methods as it has in many European countries.

TECHNIQUE

There are many different methods of giving Shiatsu, even more than in Western type massage, so the differences between therapists can be great. Here are described just a few of the basic features of Shiatsu therapy.

Treatment is usually carried out on a carpeted floor with the patient lying, or sometimes sitting, depending on the area being treated. No lubricant is used and treatment is normally given with the patient wearing loose clothing. By working on the floor it makes it more natural to use leg techniques; the knee, shin and foot are often used. The therapist is either kneeling or standing and can easily apply strong pressure when using leg techniques and can move systematically to other parts. Although one is applying pressure to a large area the treatment is aimed at acupuncture points (Tsubos) and the course of the meridians (channels) are followed. Shiatsu treatment can be painful and is considered to be more effective when it is so.

The skin and subcutaneous tissues can also be stretched with Shiatsu by moving the leg (or hand) after applying pressure or by allowing the soft tissue to glide smoothly under it, thus introducing a deep stroking action. The direction of the strokes does not always follow the direction of venous and lymphatic circulation as it does in traditional Western massage.

As well as using leg techniques to treat the arms, legs and back, the hands are also used in Shiatsu. The advantage in using the hands is that stimulation can be directed more precisely on small areas like acupuncture points.

Shiatsu has two types of effect: mechanical effects of soft tissue manipulation which induce muscular and general relaxation. There are also significant reflectory effects similar to acupuncture, which were dealt with in the previous chapter.

SHIATSU IN SPORTS MASSAGE

Shiatsu is not a rigid therapy method, but a relatively young and constantly developing art of soft tissue manipulation and stretching. It can be effectively used on sportsmen both to speed up recovery and to treat specific traumas.

16
TRIGGER POINTS

Sometimes there are painful aching areas which do not seem to respond to local treatment. Often therapists find, through general massage, remote points which refer pain to these areas. These are trigger points and are the source of the pain. If treatment is applied to these certain areas the referred pain will clear up as the tender spot disappears. Potentially every muscle can form trigger points. There are certain defined patterns where pain is referred from each muscle, although some variation exists. It is important to be aware of possible trigger points as the area where they exist may be totally symptomless. In the area where referred pain is felt muscle tension is increased and there is a tendency to form new trigger points. With a long-standing condition pain becomes gradually worse and spreads to other areas. The therapist has to search the tissues thoroughly to find hidden trigger points. Massage is the only treatment method in which this is done systematically.

The most common area to find trigger points is in the muscles, and every muscle can create several points. However, the trigger points can be found in many other tissues, not only muscles. On finding a trigger point and pressing it there is usually sharp pain radiating to the area where referred pain exists. There may also be other sensations like dull aching, the sensation of water running towards the area and warm and cold sensations, which appear later if stimulation is continued.

The pain referred from trigger points does not follow the nerve supply (it does not follow dermatome, myotome and sclerotome divisions). Stimulation of the trigger points may cause changes through the autonomic nervous system such as local excessive perspiration, hair on the skin to stand up, increase of local circulation, redness and heat. In connection with active trigger points there may be disturbance in positional and motion sensations which may cause abnormal posture and movement patterns. With tension and trigger points in the neck and masticatory muscles there may be symptoms like dizziness and blurred vision.

Trigger points can be found in:

Muscles
Fascia
Periosteum
Tendons
Ligaments
Skin
Scar Tissue

In many cases tension of some muscle bundles is revealed first when one massages through a muscle which is otherwise in normal condition. The trigger points commonly exist in these areas. This local tension increases quicker than general tension in the muscle when it is stretched and may cause pain. There is usually pain when an affected muscle is under strain. There may be a limitation in range of movement, and muscle power may be reduced although there is no atrophy. The trigger points are found as a sensitive tiny spot giving the sensation of being pricked by a needle when finger pressure is applied. Trigger points also give a sharp radiated pain to the area of referred aching. By tapping the trigger point one can cause a small local muscle twitch. When one applies steady pressure on a trigger point, sharp pain disappears first, followed by aching, in the referred area. Often the therapist notices that local muscle tension eases off at the same time. Sometimes similar effects can be obtained by pinching or stretching the skin over the trigger point, which explains why one can get positive results with connective tissue massage. This technique will be described in a later chapter.

Microscopically one will usually find no pathological changes. In cases of long-standing tension there may be nodules of contracted muscle tissue at the trigger point which may become fibrotic. This condition is sometimes called 'rheumatism' or 'myositis', which are both misleading as this is not primarily an inflammatory condition. Consequently poor results are obtained by using anti-inflammatory drugs and corticosteroids. Even poorer results are obtained with muscle relaxant medication.

There are tense muscles where one finds similar tender spots which when pressed will cause referred pain in an area that otherwise had no aching. These can be called latent trigger points. Most people have several latent trigger points which can be considered as a normal condition. In the sportsman who has many of them concentrated in a small area it means there is overstrain and increased risk of trauma.

Causes of trigger points:

Physical stress
Psychological stress
Environmental factors (cold, damp)
Trauma
Illness
Lack of rest (sleep)
Poor diet

Most of the complicated pain conditions appear to be due to a combination of several stress related factors. They affect both the physical and psychological conditions and disturb the balance of the nervous system.

When comparing the location of trigger points in relation to acupuncture points on the channels, it has been discovered that over seventy per cent have the same location. Acupuncturists also know of the existence of trigger points, but they call them Ahshi points. When extra points and Ahshi points are counted there is total overlap. Acupressure therapy in conjunction with conventional massage is the most advanced way to locate trigger points. In spite of modern technological advances, manual palpation is still the most accurate way to identify soft tissue problems.

Motor points are often confused with acupuncture and trigger points. Although there is some overlapping with these points, motor points are not part of the body's reflex mechanisms. They are often located in the middle of muscles and are areas where muscle contraction can be made most effectively with electrical devices.

Referred patterns of pain from trigger points quite often follow channels of acupuncture therapy. It is therefore unnecessary to have separate descriptions of these.

Also, this would be misleading as trigger points vary in location, and the most accurate maps are acupuncture charts. This approach allows one to look at them systematically, and thus it is easier to find the real source of the pain.

Muscles where trigger points are most likely to be found:

Head and neck
masticatory muscles
trapezius
levator scapulae
scalenus
sternocleidomastoid

Arms
extensors in lower arm

Back
infraspiratus
rhomboid muscles
erector spinae
quadratus lumborum

Front
pectoralis major and minor
rectus abdominis

Legs
tensor fasciae latae
gluteal muscles
hamstrings
triceps surae.

17
SELF MASSAGE

There are many sportsmen who try to make do with only infrequent visits to the masseur. This is often because they feel that they do not have the time or maybe they find it financially prohibitive. They may also have difficulties in finding a therapist who has experience in treating sports problems. For most sportsmen, so few treatments are not enough to be considered an integral part of a training schedule. When circumstances restrict the frequency of visits, it is still possible to get some of the benefits through self massage, although a lot will depend on the type of sport involved (for example, it is easy for a runner or footballer to massage his own legs).

Through self massage the sportsman becomes more aware of muscle tension in the treated areas. One can reduce muscle tension, and so the visits to a professional therapist will be more effective. This is because the therapist can concentrate more on problem areas and spend less time treating general tension. If the sportsman is familiar with self massage he is also able to give himself at least some treatment whenever he notices specific tension building up. It is not always possible to go straight to the therapist at the very first sign of the problem, but self massage can be performed at almost any time and place.

Self massage is also very important for the therapist who is doing hard manual work for many hours a day. He should give himself at least some treatment daily. The important parts requiring treatment are the neck, shoulders and arms. Most tension accumulates in the neck and shoulders due to isometric strain. In the arms the circulatory function will be better if they are used alternately for short periods to apply the main pressure in treatment. Working from different sides of the couch is one way of doing this, and it is a good habit to develop if one is going to manage several treatments every day. If the therapist does not give himself regular treatment, tension can build up gradually, without giving previous aching as a warning sign, until muscle strain, excessive tension or tenosynovitis develop.

The principles of self massage are the same as with normal massage treatment performed by the therapist, though not all the techniques can be applied in the same way. The techniques and basic procedures have been described in earlier chapters, and most of these can be adapted for self treatment. Similarly, specific techniques like acupressure can also be used. Before starting treatment on any part it is important to ensure it is in an unstretched and relaxed position. In this chapter we will show a basic sequence for giving self massage and demonstrate good positions for it.

The following photographs are not intended as a complete self massage programme and should be considered rather as a guideline to how it can be formed. With knowledge of the basic massage grips and how they can be used in different conditions, one has a good basis to start with. It should always be modified according to individual needs.

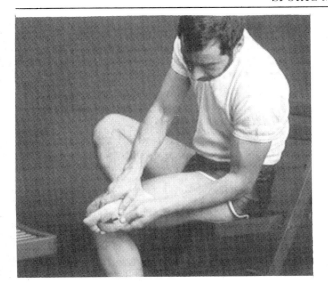
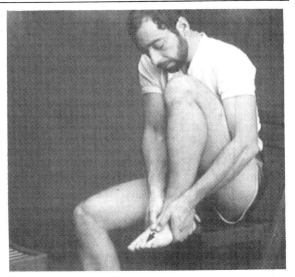
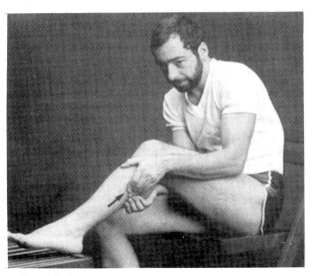
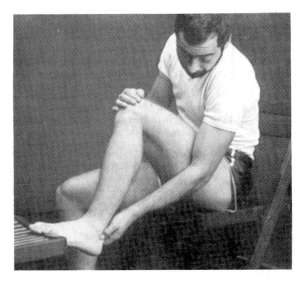

Left to right from the top:

•With the foot resting sideways on the thigh of the other leg deep longitudinal stroking can be applied along the sole of the foot, using both thumbs supporting each other. The thumbs can also be used in this position to give transverse friction to local sites of trauma

•With the knee flexed so the heel of the foot is resting on the edge of the chair. Both thumbs are used together to apply longitudinal stroking up the dorsal surface of the foot

•With the heel resting on a chair so the ankle joint is in extension and the calf muscles are relaxed. Longitudinal stroking is applied with the fingers of both hands from the heel to the back of the knee. By placing the thumbs over the shin the fingers can be squeezed into the calf muscles and deep friction can be applied to local tender areas

•With the forefoot resting on a chair so the ankle is slightly flexed and the calf muscles are lightly stretched. The fingers and thumb are used to apply deep friction to the achilles tendon

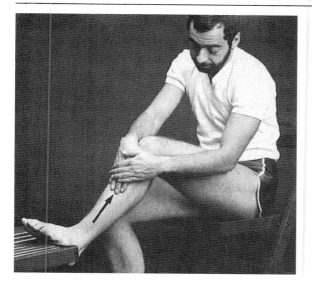
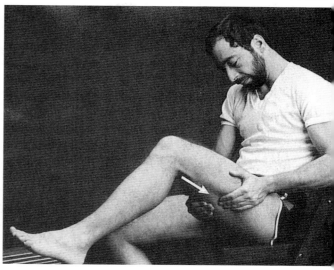
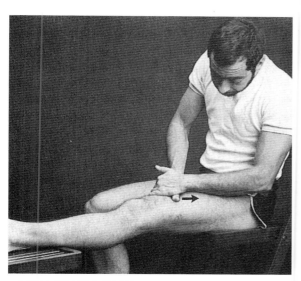
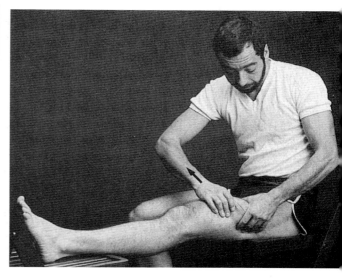

Left to right from the top:

●With the forefoot resting on a chair with the ankle in a flexed position so the shin muscles are relaxed. Longitudinal stroking is applied upwards using the fingers with the pressure reinforced with the overlying hand. It can also be done with the thumb and the overlying hand applying the force

●With the knee slightly bent and the foot resting on a chair, the hamstrings are in a relaxed position. Longitudinal stroking from knee to buttocks is applied with the fingers. It is difficult to do more than some basic stroking techniques when self treating the hamstrings, but the fingertips can be squeezed into the muscle where tender areas are felt, and transverse stroking applied

●With the leg outstretched and sitting with the back well supported – this will ensure relaxation in the thigh muscles. Deep longitudinal stroking is applied towards the inguinal area using one hand pressing down onto the fingers or thumb of the other hand

●Kneading and squeezing techniques can be applied to the quadriceps muscles in the same way as normal treatment

141

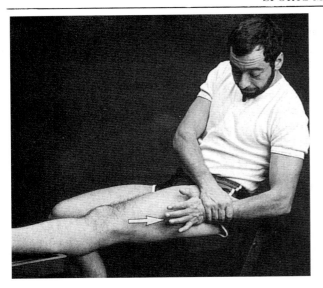

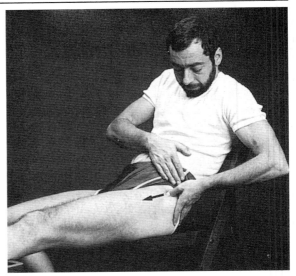

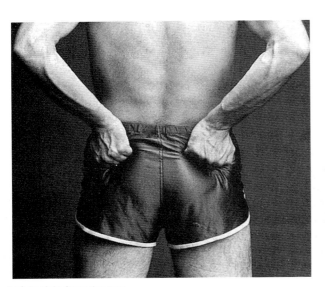

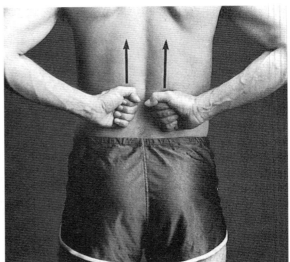

Left to right from the top:

●Longitudinal strokes are applied by using the heel of the palm with the other hand gripping the wrist and pulling inwards and reinforcing pressure up the side of the leg

●Sitting in a reclined position, deep longitudinal stroking is applied to the tensor fascia lata muscle and the attachments of the quadriceps muscle with the tips and pads of the thumb or fingers

●Standing straight with hands behind the back, rolling the knuckles of the fists is used to apply stroking to the gluteal muscles and along the iliac crest

●The radial borders of the fists are used to apply longitudinal stroking to the erector muscles of the lower back

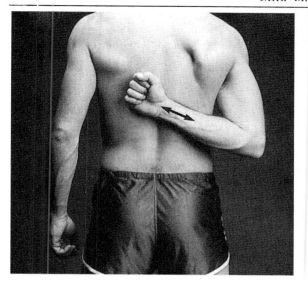
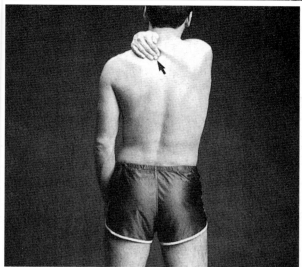
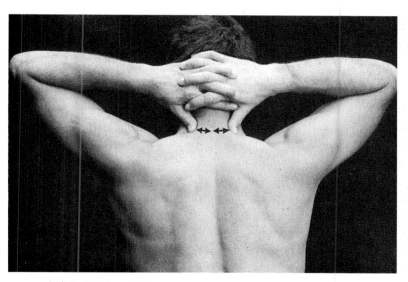
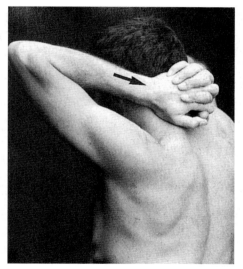

Left to right from the top:

●With the elbow flexed behind the back, the knuckles of the fist are used to apply transverse stroking to the mid back area, though it is difficult to apply much pressure

●The fingers can be used to apply transverse stroking to the shoulder muscles on the opposite side. The fingertips can be used to apply deep pressure to trigger points and friction to hard nodules

●With the fingers clasped together behind the head, the thumbs are used to apply deep stroking and friction to the upper part of the trapezius and the deeper muscles of the neck

●The palms are squeezed together to apply deep stroking and pressure to the muscles of the back of the neck -

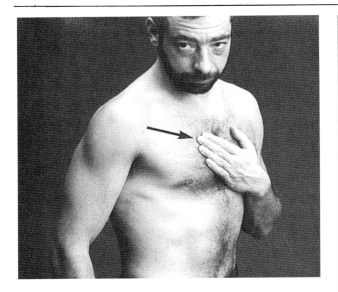

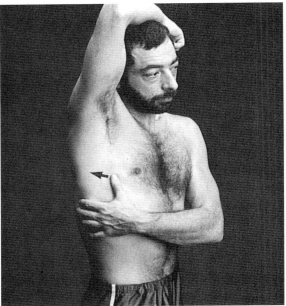

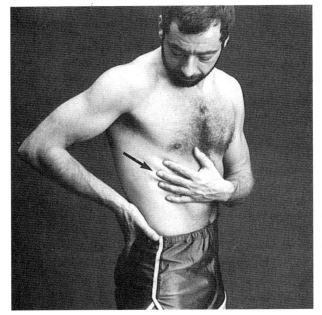

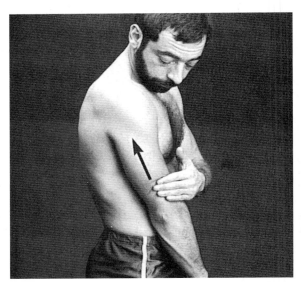

Left to right from the top:

●The fingers are used to apply longitudinal and transverse stroking to the pectoral muscles on the opposite side of the chest
●With the arm lifted up over the side of the head, deep longitudinal stroking is applied with the thumb to the seratus anterior muscle. The thumb and fingers can be used to grasp both sides of the upper part of the latissimus dorsi muscle
●With the hand placed across the chest the pads of the fingers apply stroking to the intercostal muscles
●The fingers are used to apply deep stroking on the extensor muscles of the upper arm

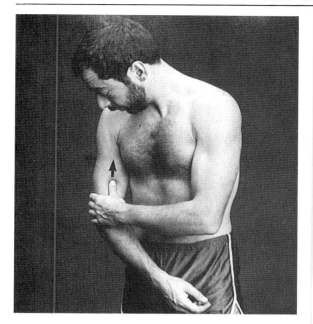

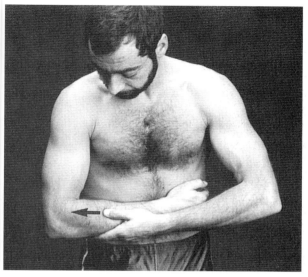

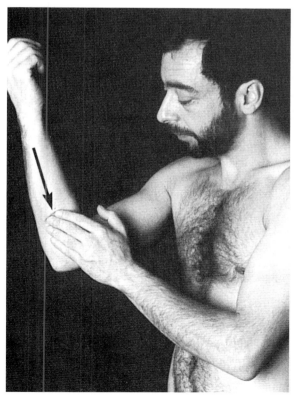

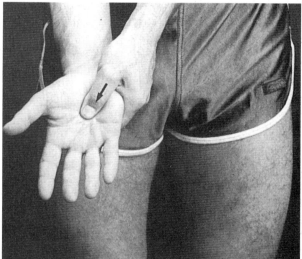

Left to right from the top:

•The thumb is used to apply deep stroking to the flexor muscles of the upper arm. The elbow should be supported in a slightly flexed position to relax the muscles
•With the elbow flexed and the forearm resting across the stomach the thumb is used to apply deep stroking to the extensor muscles of the forearm. This is vital self treatment for those prone to 'tennis elbow' conditions and for therapists doing lots of massage
•Deep longitudinal stroking applied to the flexor muscles on the forearm with the fingers
•Stroking and friction applied to the hand using the thumb

145

18
CONNECTIVE TISSUE MASSAGE (CTM)

This special massage technique was developed by a German physiotherapist, Elizabeth Dicke, in 1929. She suffered from a circulation problem of the leg which was so severe that amputation was considered. By using massage as a treatment she recovered and was able to return to work. The treatment method used by her was investigated, and it was noticed that with many internal diseases there was a change in the condition of the cutaneous tissue in local regions of the body. It was also found that by treating these affected skin areas relief was obtained in certain symptoms and diseases. This is the basis on which connective tissue therapy is formed.

Dicke published her technique first in 1953 (*Meine Bindegewebs-massage*). It has become more well known through the teachings of Maria Ebner (*Connective Tissue Manipulation*).

EFFECTS OF CTM

The treatment is aimed at the layer between the skin and muscle, that is the loose connective tissue proper. Its elasticity is dependent on several factors: location, thickness of fat layer, age, vascularity, hydration and the state of the autonomic nervous system. Increased tension in the connective tissue can be observed through the reaction of the skin. After applying finger pressure for a few seconds the depression in the skin and its pale colour will take an abnormally long time to subside.

When tension builds up in connective tissue, it loses elasticity and adhesions can form between layers which restrict its movement. The tension can cause a restriction to the fluids which need to pass through connective tissue to supply other parts like the muscles. CTM techniques release this by mechanically tearing across the layers of superficial connective tissues, so breaking any adhesions subcutaneously and causing relaxation through the reflexes.

With many painful conditions, and also with some internal diseases, there have

Basic CTM stroke: the middle finger is supported by the forefinger and the stroke is applied in an upwards direction

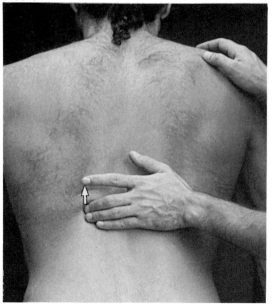

been noticed alterations in the circulation, moisture and elasticity of the skin after CTM. These changes are mainly caused via the sympathetic nervous system. With CTM, direct mechanical stretching friction is applied which causes warming, redness and sometimes swelling of the skin. These are obtained via the reflexes in the central nervous system. CTM has been shown to affect internal organs and has often helped with functional diseases and painful conditions. This is achieved mainly by balancing the sympathetic and parasympathetic nervous systems, improving circulation and inducing relaxation of the muscles.

TECHNIQUE

The person receiving treatment is usually seated. As the purpose is to cause stretching of the skin over the fascia, no oil should be used in order to obtain good contact and avoid sliding.

CTM is applied by using the tips and pads of the fingers. The middle finger is used with the forefinger to the side of it. The fingers are bent to form an angle of forty to sixty degrees with the skin. The depth of the stroke can be altered by changing the angle of the fingers to the skin; a sixty degree angle will penetrate deeper than a forty degree angle. Just enough pressure should be applied to make good contact so the skin will follow the moving fingers. Throughout the stroke the pressure and speed should remain constant. One should avoid using excessive pressure on subcutaneous structures, and the only sensation felt in the beginning of the stroke should be touch. The direction of the strokes should be radial and across the direction the fingers are pointing in. The position of the hand remains fixed and only the arm should move. An area should be treated thoroughly using overlapping strokes to cover it fully. When the technique is being carried out correctly one should experience a mild scratching or tearing sensation at the end of the stroke.

Treatment is started from the lower back, working gradually upwards. Direction of the strokes is shown in the illustrations on pp. 149–50. One moves from one part to the next after tension has been released. If there is excessive tension one should return to an area previously treated and come back to the tense part. Legs and arms are not always included in CTM treatment.

SHORT STROKES

These are carried out at right angles to bone, borders of muscle, fascia, scar tissue and adhesions. Strokes can be applied both towards and away from the structures. The first part of the stroke is to move the skin to take up the slack. Then, maintaining constant pressure, the stroke is continued for a short distance to get a stretching effect on the skin behind. At the end of the stroke the fingers are lifted off so the skin can return.

LONG STROKES

These are carried out in the same basic way as short strokes, but instead of lifting up at the end, the stroke is continued further. This is done by allowing the skinfold to run slowly and smoothly under the fingers whilst maintaining some stretch on the skin behind. Sometimes the hand, or all the finger tips running parallel, can be used; in this way a greater surface area can be covered, and better contact is made with the skin so less pressure is required. In some cases the pressure can be increased by using one hand on top of the other. Long strokes are used along muscles, tendons and bony contours.

The treatment should be continued until the loosening of tensile areas has been

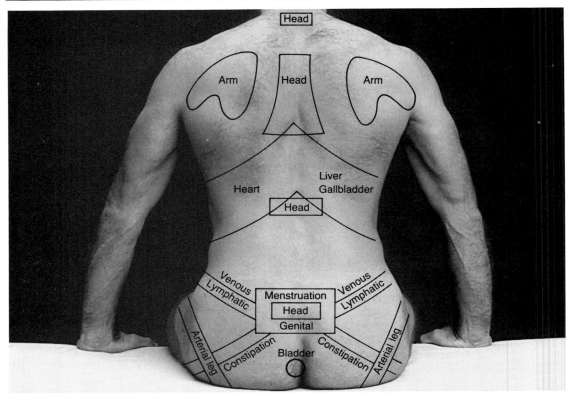

The picture shows the main reflex areas used in connective tissue massage treatment. They are not sharply defined and the areas can overlap

achieved and hypersensitive areas have disappeared. Strokes are usually repeated three to ten times. At least three strokes are required to get a proper skin reaction, and there is rarely any increase after ten.

CTM IN SPORTS MASSAGE

Excessive muscle tension

CTM can sometimes be used as a first technique where one finds muscles which are exceptionally tender and tense. In such situations the muscle can feel almost as hard as stone, making normal soft tissue massage impossible. CTM techniques applied locally can release the superficial tension and soften the muscle. Normal massage can then follow.

Relaxation

If one is accustomed to giving CTM treatment, it is possible to achieve good overall relaxation with it. This is particularly useful in sports where a high level of concentration is required.

The use of CTM in sports therapy is limited, and it should not be regarded as a complete massage treatment in itself. As the technique works only superficially it is not possible to diagnose traumas in deep structures and it cannot treat scar tissue or other deep muscle problems. However, it does offer a technique which can be effective in treating some conditions, and it is a useful addition to the skills of the sports masseur.

148

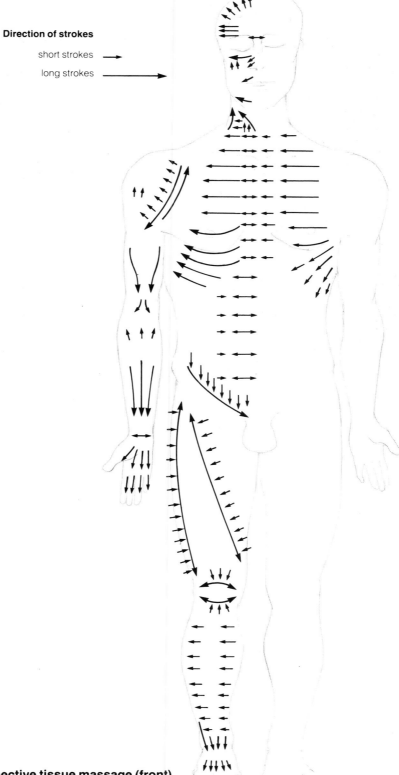

Direction of strokes

short strokes →

long strokes →

20 Connective tissue massage (front)

Direction of strokes

short strokes →

long strokes ⟶

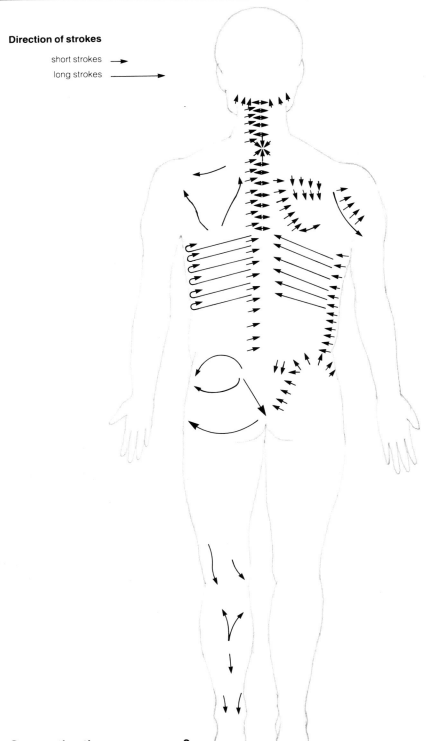

21   Connective tissue massage 2

19
LYMPH THERAPY

The fluids in healthy tissues are constantly changing. Blood rich in oxygen and nutrients is carried in the arteries and is filtrated through capillaries to the tissues. These essential ingredients are transported through cell walls and used in the cells' metabolic processes. The waste that results from metabolism is discharged into fluid that passes between cells. Most of these tissue fluids are then returned to capillaries and are transported away by the venous system. Some tissue fluid, however, is collected by lymph vessels and is transported via lymph ducts back into the central circulatory system through the left subclavian vein (see the diagram on page 21).

Lymph vessels have less pressure than blood vessels and so the circulation is slower and more easily affected by the force of gravity which it has to work against. Muscular activity is the primary motive force in the lymphatic circulation, so inactivity, sitting or standing will slow it down. Isometric muscle contraction and muscle tension will restrict the circulation. Scar tissue, especially in the area of a big lymphatic vessel, and infection of lymph ducts will further hinder the flow. The blockage of lymph flow causes swelling of the tissues, cell metabolism suffers and often pain results.

Lymph therapy aims to improve the circulation of lymph by causing a pumping and suction effect on the tissues. Lymph massage was introduced by a Danish biologist, Emil Vodder, in 1933.

TECHNIQUE

Lymph massage is performed using the pads of the fingers and thumb and/or the palms of the hands. Both hands are used alternately in a rhythmical way, with a regular increase and decrease in pressure (0 to 30 mm Hg) to create the pumping and suction effect. Circular movements are made by using the whole arm rather than just hand movements.

The therapist should always start the treatment from the lymphatic nodes in the neck, gradually moving downwards to the body and then to the limbs. Big lymph nodes should always be treated first, so when treating a limb the proximal part is worked on first before continuing downwards. This effectively clears the system of

Basic lymph therapy stroke: pressing rhythmically with the fingertips and palm of the hand combined with small rotational movements. The arrows show the two different ways of making these movements

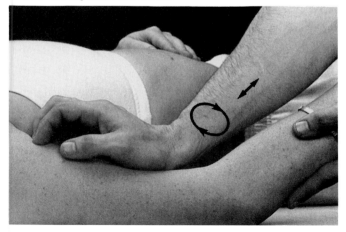

151

excess fluid and avoids stagnation which may be caused if the treatment was carried out the other way.

Contraindications to massage described in this book apply similarly to lymph therapy.

LYMPH THERAPY IN SPORTS MASSAGE

Lymph massage has been used in different kinds of odematous swelling conditions. It appears to give good results on swelling affecting the limbs after surgery and radiation therapy. Such swelling is usually due to direct damage to the circulatory system, or scar tissue hindering it. Also, swelling due to impact trauma and aseptic arthritis can be somewhat improved by lymph massage in conjunction with gentle superficial stroking on surrounding areas.

Lymph therapy is very gentle and is widely used by beauty therapists to improve circulation and elasticity of the skin. Conventional massage is more effective at treating tense muscles and scar tissue which are the most common cause of trouble for the sportsman, so lymph therapy is not often used. It is a useful technique if restricted to some special inflammatory conditions which may affect the sportsman. Lymph therapy can be applied in cases of acute trauma, other than wounds, to improve circulation in the early stage. Ordinary massage, as well as lymph therapy, can also reduce odematous swelling, and comparative studies show that there is no evidence in favour of lymph therapy.

20
ZONE THERAPY

Zone therapy (or reflexology, or reflexotherapy) originates from an old Chinese method of treating feet by massage, but it has no relationship with acupuncture. In acupuncture there is only one point of channel in the sole of the foot (Kidney 1). There are also some extra points which are rarely used because needling the sole area is very painful. In zone therapy all these areas are treated using finger pressure.

This treatment was rediscovered by Dr. William Fitzgerald in the USA who wrote a book *Zone Therapy* in 1917. It was further developed and made well known by his pupil, Eunice Ingham, who wrote a couple of books on the subject: *Stories Feet Have Told* and *Stories Feet Can Tell*. Many other people have taught massage of the feet using different names, but their maps of the different regions in the feet all originate from Ingham's maps.

THEORY

There are ten zones in man which run from the end of each toe upwards connecting with one zone running from each finger on the same side. These all reach the top of the head in different areas. In this way every part of the body has a reflectory area in the foot. The organs on the right and left sides of the body have reflex zones in the foot of the same side.

When there exists a pathological condition in a certain organ, crystals are claimed to form in the corresponding area in the foot. It is also supposed that this works in reverse. If uneven pressure is continuously caused on the feet, due for example to poor foot plant, it can cause crystals to form which can cause a pathological condition in the corresponding organ. By improving the circulation and breaking down these crystals with massage the tissues in the foot are normalised and hence the corresponding organ is treated.

The crystals claimed to be in the feet have not been shown to really exist, and in fact the therapist does not actually look for them. Instead they palpate for tender areas which are then related to certain areas according to the maps. Tenderness is assumed to suggest that a pathological condition exists in that area. This is an oversimplification of what are very complex reflexes which exist in the body. One should not consider zone therapy as a primary treatment for diseases: it has also been clearly shown in studies that reflex therapists cannot diagnose diseases by examining the feet.

TECHNIQUE

The pressure is applied with the tip of one finger, or more commonly the thumb, which is stronger, or even a knuckle can be used. One hand is used to support the foot against the working hand. Very small rotatory or screwing movements are made to add some friction to the pressure and to enable better penetration. The working hand should be changed over at regular intervals to avoid excessive strain on it. Therapists are sometimes taught to apply the technique using a bending and straightening movement with the finger; this is not advisable as it can strain the finger joints and induce arthritis (see the chapter on

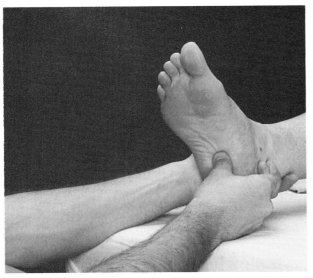

Zone therapy treatment applied with the tip of the thumb

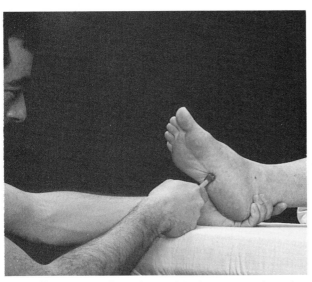

Treatment applied using a stick with a padded tip. Using tools like this requires much experience as different areas need varying amounts of pressure and sensory feedback is missing

general massage techniques). Some zone therapists use a stick with a rounded head for applying pressure. This is not recommended for the beginner who needs to first become familiar with the amount of pressure different areas need; this is more easily monitored by using the finger tip. The massaging finger should be kept almost straight, with movements carried out by the whole arm.

There is no rigid order in which massage should be applied, but all the reflectory areas mapped out in the feet should be examined systematically. Treatment should be concentrated where tender points are found. A normal treatment will last twenty to thirty minutes depending on the condition of the feet.

ZONE THERAPY IN SPORTS MASSAGE

In spite of the criticism made earlier, zone therapy can be very useful in many situations apart from just painful feet. There are painful conditions which cannot be treated with local massage, for example radicular pains in neck and lower back. Treating such areas through reflexes in the feet is safe and can often give considerable relief.

Zone therapy can also be used for functional troubles, such as abdominal pain, where it has been shown by medical examination that there is no disease. Diarrhoea and constipation caused by stress, which is often a problem with competitive sportsmen, may respond well to this treatment.

For the therapist giving sports massage, being familiar with reflexes in the feet can prove useful. While massaging the feet it takes only a little time to apply some zone therapy to selective points which relate to problem areas previously identified during treatment.

22 Zone therapy chart

This shows approximate locations of supposed
reflex areas, which may vary with each individual.

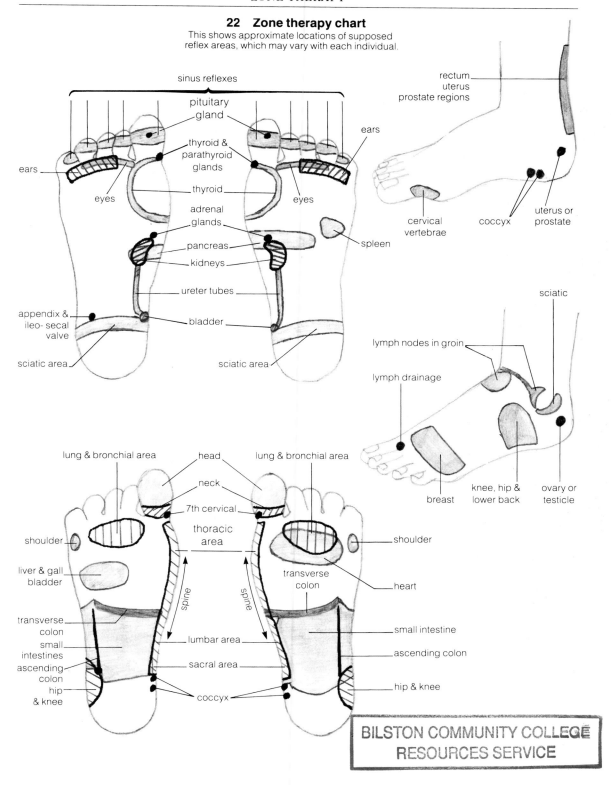

sinus reflexes

pituitary gland

ears

thyroid & parathyroid glands

ears

thyroid

eyes

eyes

adrenal glands

pancreas

spleen

kidneys

ureter tubes

appendix & ileo- secal valve

bladder

sciatic area

sciatic area

rectum
uterus
prostate regions

cervical vertebrae

coccyx

uterus or prostate

sciatic

lymph nodes in groin

lymph drainage

breast

knee, hip & lower back

ovary or testicle

lung & bronchial area

head

lung & bronchial area

neck

7th cervical

shoulder

thoracic area

shoulder

liver & gall bladder

spine

spine

heart

transverse colon

transverse colon

small intestine

small intestines

lumbar area

ascending colon

ascending colon

sacral area

hip & knee

hip & knee

coccyx

BILSTON COMMUNITY COLLEGE
RESOURCES SERVICE

BIBLIOGRAPHY

Abrahams, W. Heat versus cold therapy for treatment of muscle injuries. *Athletic training* 9:177, 1974.

Academy of Traditional Chinese Medicine, *Essentials of Chinese Acupuncture*, Peking: Foreign Languages Press, 1980.

Adams, I. The management of the injured sportsman, *Physiotherapy* 58: 6, 200, 1972.

Anderson, B. *Stretching*. London: Pelham Books, 1980.

Armour, W. *The FA Guide to the Treatment and Rehabilitation of Injuries in Sports*. Published on behalf of the Football Association, London: Heinemann, 1983.

Ashdonk, J. Arzhliche Erfahrung mit der Lymphdrainage-Massage des Krampfaderbeines. Haug Verlag, 1971.

Barr, J. and Taslitz, N. The influence of back massage on autonomic functions. *Physical Therapy* 50: 1679–1691, 1970.

Bell, A. Massage and the physiotherapist. *Physiotherapy* 50: 406–408, 1964.

Berger, M., Gerstenbrand, F. and Lewit, K. *Schmerzstudien 6, Schmerzund Bewegungssystem*, Stuttgart: Gustav Fischer, 1984.

Bernhard D. *Sports Physical Therapy*. New York: Churchill Livingstone, 1986.

Birukov, A. and Pelashov, N. Changes in psycho-physiological indices in using different techniques of sports massage. *Soviet Sports Review* 21: 1, 1986.

Bork, K., Karling, G. and Faust, G. Serum enzyme levels after 'whole body massage'. *Arch. Dermatol. Forsch.* 240: 342–348, 1971.

Calson, J. and Armour, W. *The Sports Injuries and Their Treatment*, 3rd edn. London: Century Hutchinson, 1986.

Campbell, E., Agostoni, A. and Newsom, D. *The Respiratory Muscles, Mechanics and Neural Control*. London: Lloyd-Luke, 1970.

Cash, J. *A Textbook of Medical Conditions for Physiotherapists*. London: Faber & Faber, 1976.

Chaitow, L. *Soft-Tissue Manipulation*. Thorsons, 1980.

Chamberlain, G. Cyriax's friction massage: a review. *Journal of Orthopaedic and Sports Physica Therapy* 4: 16–22, 1982.

Corbett, M. The use and abuse of massage and exercise. *Practitioner* 298: 136–139.

Cyriax, J. Deep friction massage. *Physiotherapy* 63: 60–61, 1977.

Cyriax, J. *Textbook of Orthopaedic Medicine. Vol. 2. Treatment by Manipulation, Massage and Injection*, 11th edn. London: Bailliere Tindall, 1984.

D'Ambrosia, R. *Musculoskeletal Disorders*, 2nd edn. Philadelphia: J.B. Lippincott Co., 1986.

Danneskiold-Samsoe, B., Christiansen, E., Lund, B. and Andersen, R. Regional muscle tension and pain ('fibrositis'). Effect of massage on myoglobin in plasma. *Scand J. Rehab. Med.* 15: 17–20, 1982.

Dicke, E. *Meine Bindegewebsmassage*. Stuttgart: Hippokrates Verlag, 1956.

Dubrovsky, V. Changes in muscle and venous blood flow after massage. *Soviet Sport Review* 18, 3: 134–135, 1983.

Duffin, D. Acupuncture past and present. *Physiotherapy* 64: 203–207, 1978.

Dvorak, J. and Dvorak, V. *Manual Medicine, Diagnostics*. Stuttgart: Georg Thieme Verlag, 1984.

Ebner, M. Connective tissue manipulation. *Physiotherapy* 64: 208–210, 1978.

Ebner, M. *Connective Tissue Manipulation*, 3rd edn. Florida: R.E. Krieger Publishing Co. Inc., 1985.

Feneis, H. *Pocket Atlas of Human Anatomy*. Stuttgart: Georg Thieme Verlag, 1976.

Gaymans, F. Mobilisation of the spinal column by stimulation of reflex points. *Communication from the International Symposium 'Spine and muscles'*, Prague, 1982.

Glaser, O. and Dalicho, A. *Segmentmassage*. Leipzig: Thieme Verlag, 1962.

Glover, B. and Weisenfeld, M. *The Injured Runner's Training Handbook*. New York: Penguin Books, 1985.

Goodridge, J. Muscle energy technique: definition, explanation, methods of procedure. *Journal of the American Osteopathic Association* 81: 249, 1981.

Gordon, H. Physiotherapy in muscle strains of the lower limb. *Physiotherapy* 61: 4, 102, 1975.

Grant, A. Massage with ice (cryokinetics) in the treatment of painful conditions of the musculoskeletal system. *Archives of Physical Medicine and Rehabilitation* 45: 233-238, 1964.

Grieve, G. *Modern Manual Therapy of the Vertebral Column*. New York: Churchill Livingstone, 1986.

Hagbarth, K. *Excitatory and Inhibitory Skin Areas for Flexor and Extensor Motoneurons*. Acta Physiologia Scandinavia, 1952.

Hall, T. An Analysis of Connective Tissue Massage. Proceedings of multidisciplinary international conference of manipulative therapy. Melbourne 1979: Lincoln Institute of Health Sciences, 1980.

Hansen, T. and Kristensen, J. Effect of massage, shortwave diathermy and ultrasound upon 133Xe disappearance rate from muscle and subcutaneous tissue in the human calf. *Scand. Journal Rehab. Med.* 5: 179-182, 1973.

Hartman, L. *Handbook of Osteopathic Technique*, 2nd edn. London: Hutchinson, 1985.

Hashimoto, M. *Japanese Acupuncture*. New York: Liveright Publishing Co., 1968.

Heipertz, W. Die Beeinflussung der Muskeldurshblutung durch Physiotherapeutishe Massnahmen. *Forsch. Med.* 81: 454, 1963.

Hiffa, A. *Technik der Massage*, 14th edn. Stuttgart: Ferninand Enke, 1900.

Hollis, M. *Massage for Therapists*. London: Blackwell, 1987.

Hovind, H. and Nielsen, S. Effect of massage on blood flow in skeletal muscle. *Scand. Journal Rehab. Med.* 6: 74-77, 1974.

Ingham, E. *The Stories the Feet Can Tell* and *The Stories the Feet Have Told*. Rochester, N.Y., 1959.

Janda, V. Die muskularen Hauptsyndrome bei vertebragenen Beschwerden. In *Theoretische Fortschritte und Praktische Erfahrungen der Manuellen Medizin*, p. 61. Eds., Neumann, H.

and Wolff, H. Buhl: Konkordia, 1979.

Kellgren, J. On the distribution of pain arising from deep somatic structures with charts of segmental pain areas. *Clinical Science* 4: 35, 1938.

Klafs, K. and Arnheim, D. *The Science of Sports Injury Prevention and Management. Modern principles of athletic training*, 5th edn. St. Louis: C.V. Mosby Co., 1981.

Kohlrausch, W. *Reflexzonenmassage in Muskulatur und Bindegewebe*. Stuttgart: Hippokrates Verlag, 1955.

Kottke, F. *Krujsen's Handbook of Physical Medicine and Rehabilitation*. Knapp, M., 17 *Massage*. Philadelphia: W.B. Saunders Co., 1982.

Krumhansl, B., Suction massage. *Journal of the American Physical Therapy Association* 44: 1094, 1964.

Larson, L. *Encyclopedia of Sports Sciences and Medicine*. New York: Macmillan, 1971.

Lee, J. and Warren, M. *Cold Therapy in Rehabilitation*. London: Bell & Hyman Ltd., 1978.

Leube, H. and Dicke, E. *Massage Reflektorischer Zonen im Bindegewebe*. Jena: Fischer, 1951.

Lewit, K. *Manipulative Therapy in Rehabilitation of the Locomotor System*. London: Butterworths, 1985.

Licht, E. *Massage, Manipulation and Traction*. New York: R. Krieger Publishing Co., 1976.

Ludke, H. *Technik der Massage*. Stuttgart: F. Enke Verlag, 1966.

Mann, F. *The Atlas of Acupuncture. Points and Meridians in Relation to Surface Anatomy*. London: William Heinemann Medical Books Ltd., 1967.

Masunaga, S. and Ohashi, W. *Zen Shiatsu*, 7th edn. Tokyo: Japan Publications Ltd., 1985.

Melzack, R. Myofascial trigger points: relation to acupuncture and pain, *Archives of Physical Medicine* 62: 114, 1981.

Mennell, II. *Physical Treatment by Movement Manipulation and Massage*, 5th edn. Philadelphia: The Blakiston Co., and London: J.A. Churchill Ltd., 1949.

Mitchell, F., Moran, P. and Pruzzo, N. *An Evaluation of Osteopathic Muscle Energy Procedures*. Valley Park: Pruzzo, 1979.

Moore, K. *Clinically Orientated Anatomy*, 2nd edn. Baltimore: Williams & Wilkins, 1985.

Muller, E. and Esch, J. Die Wirkung der Massage aug die Leistungsfahigkeit von Muskein. *Int. Z. Angew. Physiol.* 22: 240, 1966.

Nordschow, M. and Bierman, W. The influence of manual massage on muscle relaxation: effect on trunk flexion. *Journal of the American Physical Therapy Association* 42: 653-657, 1962.

Ohashi, W. *Shiatshu. Do-it-yourself*, 5th edn. London: Unwin Paperbacks, 1984.

Peterson, L. and Renstrom, P. *Sports Injuries. Their Prevention and treatment.* London: Dunitz Ltd., 1986.

Read, M. *Sports Injuries.* London: Breslich & Foss, 1984.

Reily, T. *Sports Fitness and Sports Injuries.* London: Faber & Faber Ltd., 1981.

Richens, C. and Brizzee, K. Effects of cutaneous stimulation on circulation, duodenal arterioles and capillary beds. *Journal of Neurophysiology* 12: 131-137, 1979.

Rolf, I. *Rolfing: The Interpretation of Human Structures.* New York: Harper & Row, 1978.

Schmidt, K. Das Verhalten der elektrischen Muskelaktivitat nach maschineller Vibrationsmassage. *Deutsche medizinishe Wochenschrift* 93: 114-116, 1968.

Sedlacek, E. Fusszonenmassage. *Archiv fur Physikalische Therapie* 19: 373-375, 1967.

Serizawa, K. *Effective Tsubo Therapy. Simple and Natural Relief Without Drugs.* Tokyo: Japan Publications Inc., 1984.

Simons, D. and Travell, J. Myofascial origin of low back pain. *Postgraduate Medicine* 73: 66, 1983.

Solveborn, S.A. *The Book about Stretching.* Japan Publications Inc., 1985.

Stoddard, A. *Manual of Osteopathic Technique*, 10th edn. London: Hutchinson, 1978.

Storms, H. Diagnostic and therapeutic massage. *Archives of Physical Medicine* 25, 1944.

Tappan, F. *Healing Massage Techniques. A Study of Eastern and Western Methods.* Virginia: Reston Publishing Co. Inc. 1978.

Travell, H. and Simons, D. *Myofascial Pain and Dysfunction. The Trigger Point Manual.* Baltimore: Williams & Wilkins, 1983.

Wakim, K. The effects of massage on the circulation in normal and paralysed extremities. *Archives of Physical Medicine* 30: 135, 1949.

Wakim, K. Influence of centripetal rhythmic compression on localised oedema of an extremity. *Archives of Physical Medicine* 36: 98, 1955.

Walker, II. Deep transverse frictions in ligament healing. *Journal of Orthopaedic and Sports Physical Therapy* 6: 89-94, 1984.

Watson, J. Pain mechanisms, a review. *Australian Journal of Physiotherapy* 27: 135-143, 1981.

Waylonis, G. The physiologic effects of ice massage. *Archives of Physical Medicine and Rehabilitation* 48: 37-42, 1967.

Wensel, L. *Acupuncture in Medical Practice.* Virginia: Reston Publishing Co., 1980.

Williams, J. and Sperryn, P. *Sports Medicine. E.* London: Arnold Publishers Ltd., 1976.

Williams, P. and Warwick R. *Gray's Anatomy*, 36th edn. Edinburgh: Churchill Livingstone, 1980.

Wood, E. and Becker, P. *Beard's Massage*, 3rd edn. Philadelphia: W.B. Saunders Co., 1981.

Wright, H., Korr, I. and Thomas, P. Local and regional variations in cutaneous vasomotor tone of the human trunk. *Acta Neurovegetativa* 22: 33, 1960.

Xi-zhen, C. *The Massotherapy of Traditional Chinese Medicine.* Hongkong: Hai Feng Publishing Co., 1985.

GLOSSARY

Abductor. Any muscle which moves one part of the body away from another or away from the midline of the body.

Acromion. An oblong process at the top of the spine of the scapula.

Acute. Of rapid onset with severe intense symptoms.

Adductor. Any muscle that moves one part of the body towards another or towards the midline of the body.

Adhesion. The joining of two normally separate tissues by fibrous connective tissue.

Alkalosis. A condition in which the alkaline level in body fluids is abnormally high.

Annular (ligament). A ring shaped ligament around the radius connecting it to the ulna bone.

Antagonist. A muscle whose action opposes that of another muscle.

Anterior. Relating to the front part of the body, limb or organ.

Aorta. The main artery of the body.

Aponeurosis. A strong fibrous tissue that replaces a tendon in muscles that have multiple attachments close together.

Arcus. An arch.

Artery. Blood vessel carrying blood away from the heart.

Arteriole. Small branch of an artery.

Atrophy. The wasting away of an organ or tissue.

Auricle. The flap of skin and cartilage of the external ear.

Axilla. The armpit.

Axon. Part of the nerve which carries impulses away from nerve cells.

Body Image. A cognative self awareness of parts of the body.

Brachial. Relating to the arm.

Bursa. A small sack of connective tissue, lined with synovial membrane and containing fluid (synovia). They help reduce friction and are normally found around joints where ligaments and tendons pass over bones.

Calcaneus. Heel bone.

Canthus. Either corner of the eye.

Capillary. An extremely narrow blood vessel.

Capsulitis. Inflammation of the connective tissue capsule surrounding a joint.

Carotid artery. Either of the two main arteries in the neck.

Carpal. The bones of the wrist.

Cartilage (hyaline). A dense connective tissue layer found on the surface of the bones in joints as well as several other areas.

Cervical vertebrae (C1-7). The bones making up the neck region of the spine.

Clavicle. The collar bone.

Coccyx. The lowest part of the spine.

Collagen. A relatively inelastic protein with high tensile strength being an important part of the tendon structure.

Collateral (ligament). Ligament on the side of a joint.

Condyle. A rounded protuberence that occurs on some bones.

Coracoid process. A process that curves forwards from the top front side of the scapula.

Cortex. Outer part of an organ.

Corticosteroid. A steriod hormone released by the adrenal cortex.

Costal. Relating to the ribs.

Crepitus. A crackling sound or grating feeling produced between tendon and tendon sheath or by bone rubbing on bone or roughened cartilage.

Crural. Relating to the leg.

Cubital. Relating to the elbow or forearm.

Cuneiform bones. Three bones in tarsus of the foot.

Cutaneous. Relating to the skin.

Dermatome. A certain part of the central nervous system (nerve root) innervating a certain part of skin.

Distal. Situated away from something.

Dorsal. Relating to the back part of the body, limb or organ.

Dorsiflexion. Flexion of the foot upwards, or the hand in an opposite direction to the palmer side.

Efferent. Nerves that convey impulses away from the brain or spinal cord.

Endorphin. A group of chemical compounds that occur naturally in the brain and are shown to have pain relieving properties.

Enzyme. A protein that speeds up the rate of chemical reaction.

Epicondyle. The protuberance above the condyle of the bone.

Epigastrium. The upper central region of the abdomen.

Erysipelas. A bacterial infection of the skin and underlying tissues.

Extension. The straightening of a limb or other part.

Extensor. A muscle that causes the straightening of a limb or other part.

Facet. A flat area making an articular surface for example in the vertebral bones.

Fascia. A superficial membrane surrounding the body just beneath the skin. Deeper fascia surrounds muscle groups and individual muscles.

Femur. Thigh bone.

Fibrosis. Thickening and scarring of connective tissue.

Flexion. The bending of a joint so that the bones forming it are brought towards each other.

Flexor. Any muscle that causes bending of a limb or other part.

Foramen. An opening or hole.

Fossa iliac. The hollow area on the inner surface of the ilium bone.

Haematoma. An accumulation of blood within the tissues that clots to form a solid swelling.

Hamate. A hook shaped bone of the wrist.

Hiatus. An opening or aperture.

Histamine. An inflammation causing enzyme.

Humerus. The bone of the upper arm.

Iliac. Relating to the hip.

Ilium. A wide bone forming the upper part of each side of the hip bone.

Inferior. Lower in relation to another structure.

Infra-. Prefix denoting 'below'.

Inguinal. Relating to the region of the groin.

Interosseus membrane. A fibrous structure between two bones.

Ischaemia. A deficient flow of blood to a part of the body.

Ischium. The bone forming the lower part of the hip bone.

Isometric. When a muscle contracts but despite an increase in tension does not shorten or lengthen.

-itis. Suffix denoting inflammation.

Kyphosis. Excessive outward curvature of the spine, causing a hunching of the back.

Lactic acid. A product that forms in the cells as the end product of energy metabolism in the absence of oxygen.

Lateral. Situated at the side.

Ligament. A tough band of fibrous connective tissue that links two bones together at a joint. Ligaments are inelastic but flexible, limiting movement of the joint in certain directions.

Longitudinal. Along the line the fibres run in.

Lordosis. Excessive inward curvature of the spine causing 'sway-back' and 'hump-back'.

Lumbar vertebrae (L1-5). The bones of the spine, in the lower part of the back.

Lumbo-. Prefix denoting the lumbar region.

Lymph. A fluid present in the vessels of the lymphatic system that bathes the tissues.

Malleolus. Either of the two protuberences on each side of the ankle.

Mamilla. The nipple.

Mechanoreceptor. A group of cells that respond to mechanical distortion such as that caused by stretching or compressing a tissue, by generating a nerve impulse in a sensory nerve.

Medial. Relating to or situated in the central region of a tissue, organ or the body.

Mandible. The lower jawbone.

Mastoid. The process of the temporal bone.

Meniscus. A crescent shaped structure, such as a fibro cartilage disc stabilising a synovial joint.

Metabolism. The sum of all the chemical changes that take place within the cell of the body.

Metacarpal. The bones of the hand.

Myositis. Inflammation of a muscle.

Myotome. A certain part of the central nervous system (nerve root) innervating a certain part of muscle.

Necrosis. Death of the tissue.

Occipital bone. A bone forming the back of the skull and the base of the cranium.

Oedema. Excessive accumulation of fluid in the body tissues.

Oesophogus. The gullet: a muscular tube which extends from the pharynx to the stomach.

Olecranon process. The large process in the proximal part of the ulna in the elbow joint.

Orbit. The cavity in the skull that contains the eye.

Ossification. The formation of bone.

Palpate. To examine by careful feeling with the hands and fingertips.

Passive movements. Movements induced by another person without one's own effort.

Parietal bones. The two bones forming the top of the skull.

Patella. Kneecap.

Periosteum. A layer of dense connective tissue that covers the surface of a bone except at the articular surfaces.

Peristalsis. A wavelike involuntary movement that progresses along some of the hollow tubes of the body, for example the intestines.

Phalanges. The bones of the fingers and toes.

Pisiform. The smallest bone of the wrist.

Plantar. Relating to the sole of the foot.

Plexus. A network of nerves.

Popliteal. Relating to the space at the back of the knee.

Postural muscles. Muscles that serve to maintain the upright posture of the body against the force of gravity.

Prolapse. The displacement of a tissue through another tissue.

Pronate. Turning the foot so that the sole faces outwards (ankle rolls inwards), or turning the hand so the palm faces downwards.

Proximal. Situated close to something.

Radial. Relating to or associated with the radius.

Radius. The outer and shorter bone of the forearm.

Retinaculum. A thickened band of connective tissue which acts to hold various tissues in place.

Sacrum. A triangular part of the spine consisting of five fused vertebrae forming the midpart of the pelvis.

Sacro-. Prefix denoting to the sacrum.

Scaphoid. A boat shaped bone of the wrist.

Scapula. The shoulder blade.

Scar. Any mark left after the healing of a wound, where the damaged tissues fail to repair fully and are replaced by fibrous connective tissue.

Sclerotome. A certain part of the central nervous system (nerve root) innervating a certain part of bone.

Scoliosis. A lateral (sideways) deviation of the spine.

Sheath. A thin layer of connective tissue that envelopes a structure.

Sprain. Injury to a ligament caused by sudden overstretching.

Sternum. The breastbone.

Strain. Excessive overload or stretching of a muscle or tendon.

Styloid process. Spiny projection from bone.

Supinate. Turning the foot so the sole faces inwards, or turning the hand palm upwards.

Supra-. Prefix denoting 'above'.

Symphysis pubis. The joint between the pubic bones of the pelvis.

Synovial joint. A freely moveable joint which is surrounded by a synovial capsule containing fluid which provides lubrication.

Tarsal bones. The bones of the foot.

Temporal bone. Either of a pair of bones of the cranium forming part of the side and base of the skull.

Tendon. A tough whitish cord consisting of many parallel bundles of collagen fibres that serve to attach muscle to bone.

Teno-. Prefix denoting a tendon.

Tenosynovitis. Inflammation of a tendon sheath.

Thoracic vertebrae (Th1-12). The bones of the

spine to which the ribs are attached.

Thyroid gland. A large endocrine gland below the thyroid cartilage in the front of the neck.

Tibia. The shin bone. The inner and larger bone of the lower leg.

Tonus (tone). The state of contraction of a muscle without any voluntary effort.

Tragus. The projection of cartilage in the outer ear.

Transverse. Across the direction the fibres run in.

Trapezium. A bone of the wrist.

Trauma. A physical wound or injury.

Trochanter. The protuberance found at bone.

Tuberosity. A large rounded formation of bone.

Ulna. The inner and longer bone of the forearm.

Umbilicus. The navel.

Valgus. A deformity that displaces the knees towards the midline and the foot away from the midline.

Varus. A deformity that displaces the knees away from the midline and the foot towards the midline.

Vertebrae. The bones which comprise the spine.

Vasoactive. Affecting the diameter of blood vessels, especially arteries.

Vein. A blood vessel carrying blood towards the heart.

Vena cava. Either of two main veins conveying blood from other veins to the heart.

Vessel. A tube conveying body fluid.

Zygomatic (malar) bone. The bone that forms the prominent part of the cheeks.

INDEX